The Complete Fertility Diet

Cookbook for Men

2000 Days Delicious Recipes to Improve Male Reproductive Health System | Meals to Boost Sperm Quality

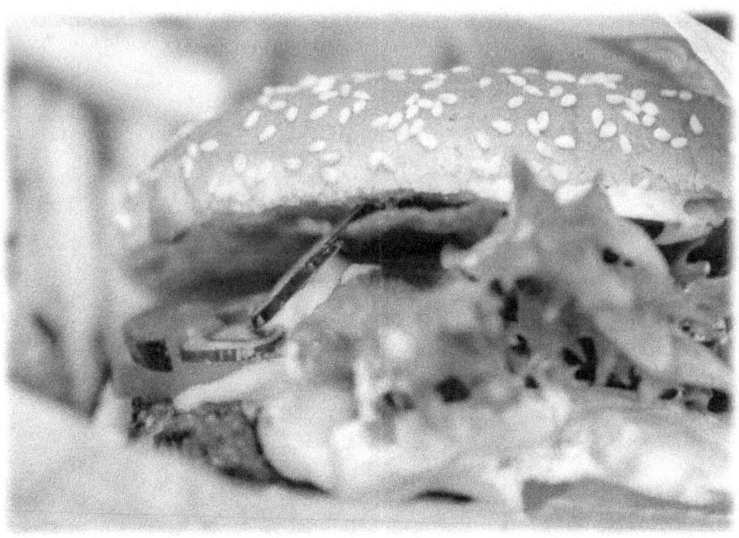

Eric A. Randell

COPYRIGHT

No part of this book may be reproduced in written, electronic, recording, or photocopying without the permission of the publisher or author.
The exception would be in the case of brief quotations embodied in the critical articles or reviews and pages where permission is specifically granted by the publisher or author.
Although every precaution has been taken to verify the accuracy of the information contained herein, the author and publisher assume responsibility for any errors or omissions. No liability is assumed for damages that may result from the use of the information contained within.
All Right Reserved©2023

GAIN ACCESS TO MORE BOOKS FROM ME

TABLE OF CONTENTS

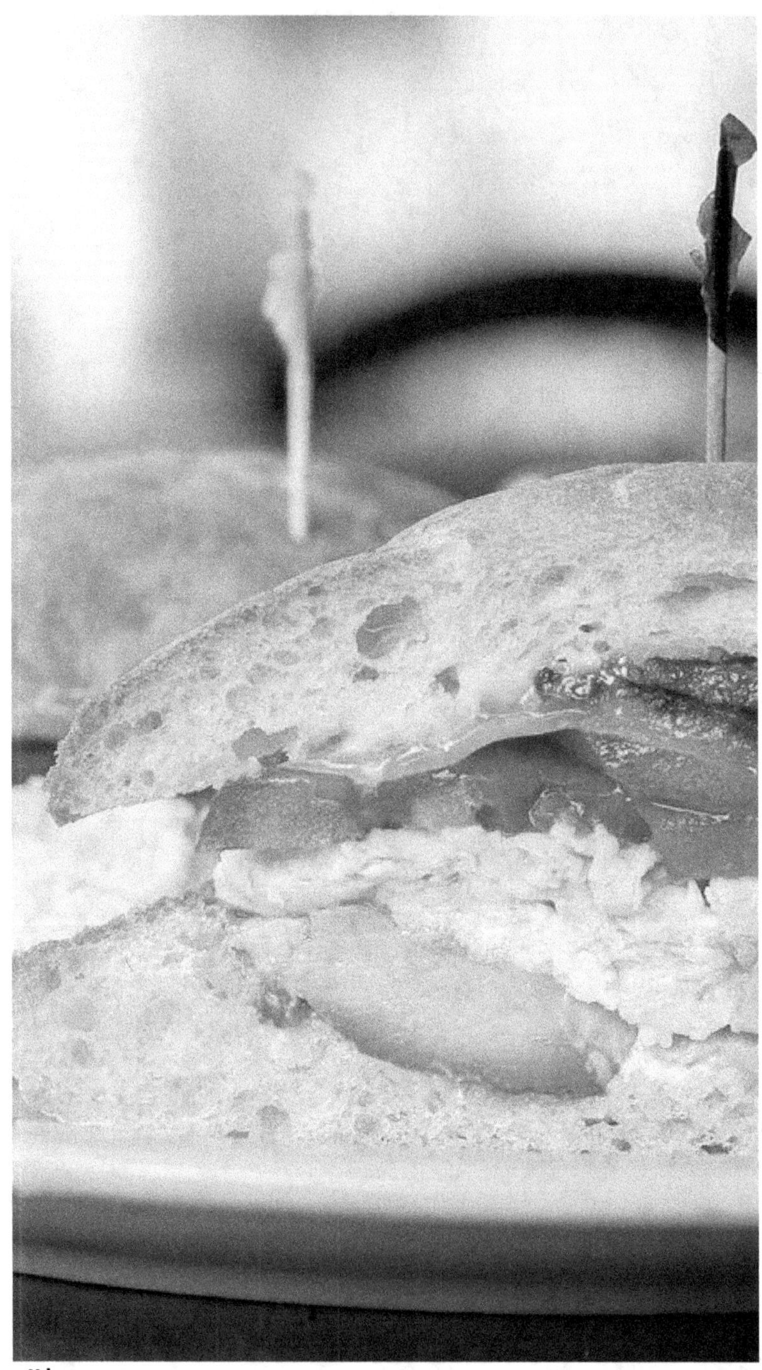

INTRODUCTION

In the heartrending journey of struggling with infertility, a couple battled years of emotional turmoil. For over three years, their desperate desire for a child cast shadows on their once harmonious marriage. The weight of unfulfilled dreams led to conflicts and sorrow, straining their relationship to its limits. In their pursuit of hope, they turned to unconventional yet life-changing solutions: Fertility Diet Cookbooks. Determined to overcome infertility, the man sought guidance from a Fertility Diet Cookbook for Men, while his wife explored the insights within a _women's Fertility Cookbook_. Together, they embraced excrcises, dietary changes, and lifestyle adjustments recommended in these guides.

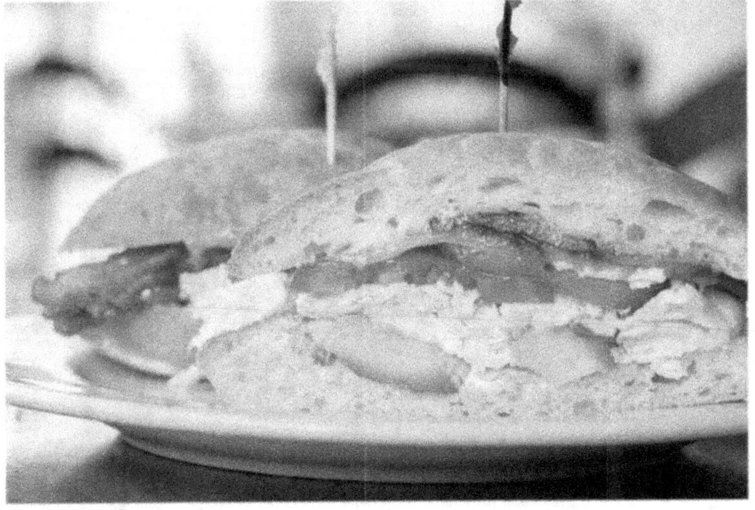

Miraculously, their unwavering commitment bore fruit. Their lives transformed as they found themselves on the path to parenthood. The healing power of these Cookbooks not only mended their relationship but also granted them the gift of a cherished child. Their fervent advice echoes loud and clear: every couple as well as singles, regardless of their fertility struggles, should embrace the wisdom of a fertility Cookbook. These resources, often overlooked, offer invaluable guidance, exercises, and dietary plans that can pave the way toward overcoming infertility issues.

The importance of fertility Cookbooks cannot be overstated. They provide a roadmap, offering hope and practical solutions to couples navigating the tumultuous waters of infertility. Their experience stands as a testament to the transformative impact of these resources, urging everyone to explore this invaluable aid to avoid or resolve fertility challenges. *Click here for pregnancy cookbook*

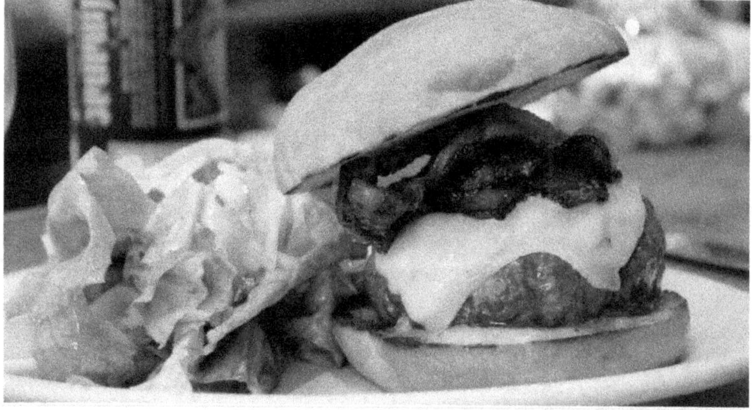

Ways to Increase Men's Fertility

1. Engage in regular physical activity

Regular exercise can not only benefit overall health but also contribute to enhanced fertility by elevating testosterone levels and semen quality. Studies have demonstrated that men who engage in regular physical activity tend to have higher testosterone levels and better semen quality compared to those who are inactive. Nevertheless, it's important to note that excessive exercise can have an adverse effect and potentially decrease testosterone levels, so maintaining a proper balance is crucial. Additionally, ensuring sufficient zinc intake can help mitigate the risk of lowered testosterone levels associated with excessive exercise.

2. Consume adequate vitamin C

Vitamin C is well-known for its immune-boosting properties, and it may also play a role in improving fertility. Research suggests that taking antioxidant supplements, such as vitamin C, could be beneficial for fertility. A study involving infertile men found that taking 1,000-mg vitamin C supplements twice daily for up to 2 months resulted in a 92% increase in sperm motility, a more than 100% increase in sperm count, and a 55% reduction in the proportion of deformed sperm cells. Furthermore, it was observed that vitamin C supplements significantly enhanced sperm count and motility, while decreasing the number of deformed sperm cells.

3. Adopt relaxation techniques and manage stress

In addition to impacting your mood, stress may have negative effects on sexual satisfaction and fertility. Research suggests that the hormone cortisol plays a role in how stress affects fertility. Prolonged stress can elevate cortisol levels, which can in turn have detrimental effects on testosterone. When cortisol levels rise, testosterone levels often decline. Therefore, managing stress can be vital to fertility, and simple activities such as spending time in nature, meditating, exercising, or socializing can help reduce stress levels.

4. Ensure adequate vitamin D intake

Vitamin D is essential for both male and female fertility and can also potentially enhance testosterone levels. Research has shown that men with vitamin-D deficiency are more likely to have low testosterone levels, and a controlled study demonstrated that supplementing with 3,000 IU of vitamin D3 daily for a year raised testosterone levels by approximately 25%.

5. Maintain optimal zinc levels

Zinc, an essential mineral abundant in animal foods, plays a crucial role in male fertility. Studies have linked low zinc levels or deficiency to reduced testosterone, poor sperm quality, and an increased risk of male infertility. Furthermore, zinc supplements may help counteract decreased testosterone levels associated with excessive high-intensity exercise.

6. Consider maca root supplements

Incorporating maca root supplements into your diet may enhance libido, fertility, and sexual performance. Native to central Peru, maca root has a history of traditional use for its libido-boosting and fertility-enhancing properties. Research has indicated that consuming 1.5 -- 3 grams of dried maca root for up to 3 months improved self-reported sexual desire. Additionally, studies have suggested that maca root may improve sexual performance, with findings showing slight improvements in erectile function and sexual well-being in men with mild erectile dysfunction after taking 2.4 grams of dried maca root for 12 weeks.

Foods to Avoid for Male Fertility

Male fertility issues can be a source of frustration for couples trying to conceive, as it not only affects physical health but also takes a toll on mental and emotional well-being. However, one way to address and potentially improve fertility is by examining our diet. The foods we consume play a significant role in determining fertility levels.

1. **Soy Products:** While soy products are generally considered healthy, they may not be the best choice for men trying to conceive. Soy contains isoflavones, which have an estrogenic effect. This can lead to increased estrogen levels in the body and a subsequent decrease in testosterone levels. Lower testosterone levels can have a negative impact on sperm quality and count, hindering healthy fertility in men.

2. **Processed Meats:** Processed meats, such as ham, pepperoni, sausages, bacon, and salami, should be consumed in moderation or avoided altogether. Research has shown that excessive consumption of processed meats can result in a decreased sperm count and reduce sperm quality by up to 23 percent. Furthermore, men who consume a significant amount of processed meats tend to have a higher percentage

of abnormally shaped sperm, which can make it more difficult to conceive.

3. Fish with High Mercury Levels: Certain fish, like swordfish, tuna, and tilefish, contain high levels of mercury. As predators, these fish consume other smaller fish, leading to an accumulation of mercury. Mercury is toxic and consuming these types of fish in large quantities can have negative effects on the reproductive system, potentially causing fertility issues.

4. Carbonated Drinks: Carbonated drinks, colas, and energy drinks can also impact male fertility. Drinking a quart of carbonated drinks daily can reduce sperm count by 30 percent and significantly decrease sperm motility. Additionally, these beverages often have high sugar content, which can increase oxidative stress in the body, further damaging sperm DNA.

5. Canned and Tinned Foods: Canned and tinned foods, which contain the compound Bisphenol (BPA), should be minimized. BPA mimics estrogen in the human body, similar to excess soy consumption. This can lead to a drop in testosterone levels and adversely affect sperm quality. It is advisable to avoid canned fruits and foods as much as possible.

6. High-Fat Dairy Products: High-fat dairy products like cheese and full-cream milk may also negatively impact male reproductive health. Recent studies suggest that these products can significantly decrease sperm motility and count. Additionally, full-fat dairy products may contain residues of medications given to cows, which can further affect the reproductive system.

7. Trans Fats: Consuming high amounts of trans fat, found in baked and fried foods like cakes, cookies, pies, biscuits, fried chicken, and French fries, is linked to a reduction in total sperm count. Excessive consumption of these foods not only affects overall health but also increases the risk of obesity. Obesity is a major cause of fertility issues in males.

8. Alcohol: Regular alcohol consumption can deteriorate overall health and significantly impact reproductive health in both genders. Excessive alcohol intake often leads to fertility problems in men, such as low sperm count, low testosterone levels, and erectile dysfunction. Additionally, the dehydrating effects of alcohol can worsen underlying health problems. It is advisable to limit or avoid alcohol consumption to boost fertility.

Paying attention to your diet is crucial for a healthy reproductive system and fertility. Avoiding or moderating the consumption of soy products, processed meats, fish high in mercury, carbonated drinks, canned foods, high-fat dairy products, trans fats, and alcohol can potentially improve male fertility and increase the chances of successful conception.

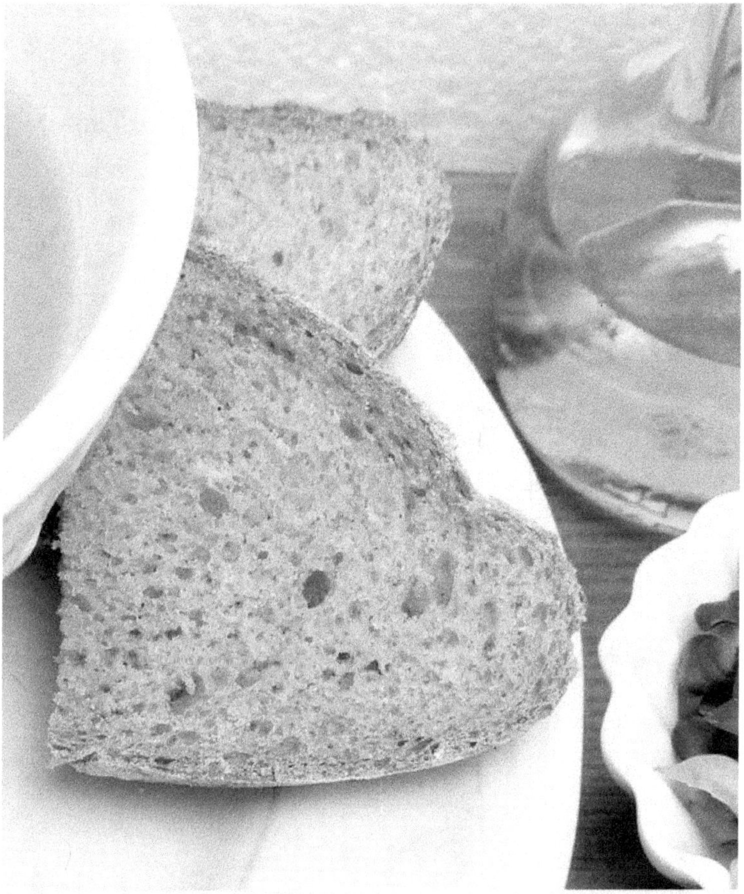

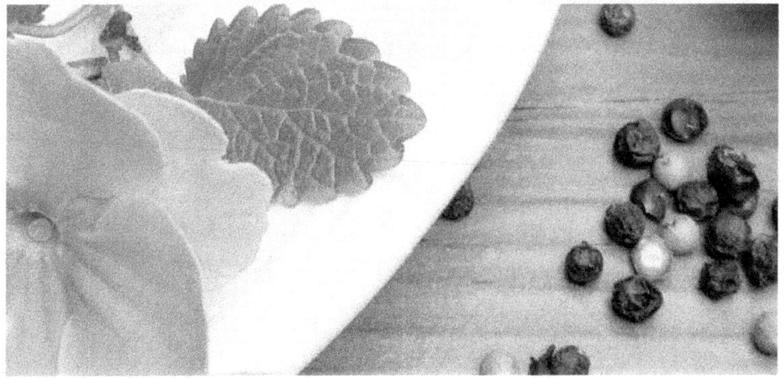

BREAKFAST RECIPES

Power-Packed Oatmeal Bow

Servings: 2 | Prep Time: 5 mins | Cooking Time: 10 mins

Ingredients:

- 1 cup rolled oats
- 2 cups milk (of your choice)
- 1 banana, sliced
- 1 tablespoon honey
- 1/4 cup chopped walnuts

Instructions:

- ✓ In a saucepan, put together the oats and milk. Cook over moderate to high heat until creamy.
- ✓ Serve in a bowl, top with banana slices, drizzle honey, and sprinkle walnuts.

Spinach and Tomato Scramble

Servings: 2 | Prep Time: 5 mins | Cooking Time: 10 mins

Ingredients:

- 4 large eggs
- 1 cup fresh spinach leaves
- 1/2 cup diced tomatoes

- 1/4 cup shredded cheddar cheese
- Salt and pepper to taste

Instructions:

- ✓ Whisk eggs in a bowl and adjust with a little salt and pepper.
- ✓ Heat a non-stick skillet over moderate to high temperature, add spinach and tomatoes, cook for two minutes.
- ✓ Pour in the eggs and cook until they start to set, then sprinkle cheese on top.
- ✓ Stir until eggs are fully cooked. Serve hot.

Avocado Toast Delight

Servings: 2 | Prep Time: 5 mins | Cooking Time: 5 mins

Ingredients:

- 2 slices of whole-grain bread
- 1 ripe avocado
- 1/2 lemon, juiced
- Salt and pepper to taste
- Red pepper flakes (optional)

Instructions:

- ✓ Toast the bread until golden brown.
- ✓ Mash the avocado with lemon juice, salt, and pepper.
- ✓ Spread the avocado mixture on the toast and sprinkle with red pepper flakes if desired.

Greek Yogurt Parfait

Servings: 2 | Prep Time: 5 mins | Cooking Time: 0 mins

Ingredients:

- 1 cup Greek yogurt
- 1/2 cup mixed berries
- 2 tablespoons honey
- 1/4 cup granola

Instructions:

- ✓ In a glass, layer Greek yogurt, berries, honey, and granola.
- ✓ Repeat the layers. Serve chilled.

Banana and Almond Smoothie

Servings: 2 | Prep Time: 5 mins | Cooking Time: 0 mins

Ingredients:

- 2 ripe bananas
- 1 cup almond milk
- 1/4 cup almond butter
- 1 tablespoon honey
- Ice cubes

Instructions:

- ✓ Blend bananas, almond milk, almond butter, honey, and ice until smooth.
- ✓ Transfer into glasses and serve immediately.

Veggie Breakfast Burrito

Servings: 2 | Prep Time: 10 mins | Cooking Time: 15 mins

Ingredients:

- 4 large eggs
- 1/2 bell pepper, diced
- 1/2 onion, chopped
- 1/2 cup black beans

- 1/2 cup shredded cheese
- 4 whole-grain tortillas

Instructions:

- ✓ Scramble eggs in a pan, then set aside.
- ✓ Sauté bell pepper and onion until soft, then add black beans.
- ✓ Fill tortillas with eggs, vegetable mixture, and cheese.
- ✓ Roll them up and heat in a pan until the cheese melts.

Peanut Butter and Banana Pancakes

Servings: 4 | Prep Time: 10 mins | Cooking Time: 15 mins

Ingredients:

- 1 cup whole wheat flour
- 2 teaspoons baking powder
- 1/4 teaspoon salt
- 1 cup milk
- 1 ripe banana, mashed
- 2 tablespoons peanut butter
- 1 egg
- 2 tablespoons honey

Instructions:

- ✓ In a bowl, mix flour, baking powder, and salt.
- ✓ In another bowl, whisk together milk, banana, peanut butter, egg, and honey.
- ✓ Put together wet and dry ingredients and stir until smooth.
- ✓ Cook pancake batter on a griddle until golden brown.

Sweet Potato Hash

Servings: 2 | Prep Time: 10 mins | Cooking Time: 20 mins

Ingredients:

- 2 sweet potatoes, peeled and diced
- 1/2 onion, chopped
- 1 red bell pepper, diced
- 2 tablespoons olive oil
- 1 teaspoon paprika
- Salt and pepper to taste

Instructions:

- ✓ Heat olive oil in a pan, add sweet potatoes, onion, and bell pepper.
- ✓ Sprinkle with paprika, salt, and pepper.

✓ Cook until sweet potatoes are tender and slightly crispy.

Quinoa Breakfast Bowl

Servings: 2 | Prep Time: 10 mins | Cooking Time: 0 mins

Ingredients:

- 1 cup cooked quinoa
- 1/2 cup Greek yogurt
- 1/4 cup mixed berries
- 2 tablespoons honey
- 1/4 cup chopped almonds

Instructions:

✓ In a bowl, layer quinoa, Greek yogurt, berries, honey, and almonds.

✓ Repeat the layers. Serve chilled.

Veggie Omelet

Servings: 2 | Prep Time: 10 mins | Cooking Time: 10 mins

Ingredients:

- 4 large eggs
- 1/2 cup diced bell peppers
- 1/4 cup diced tomatoes
- 1/4 cup chopped spinach
- 1/4 cup shredded mozzarella cheese
- Salt and pepper to taste

Instructions:

- ✓ Whisk eggs in a bowl and adjust with a little salt and pepper.
- ✓ Pour eggs into a hot, greased pan.
- ✓ Add peppers, tomatoes, and spinach.
- ✓ Once the omelet sets, sprinkle cheese and fold in half.

Blueberry Banana Smoothie Bowl

Servings: 2 | Prep Time: 5 mins | Cooking Time: 0 mins

Ingredients:

- 2 ripe bananas
- 1 cup frozen blueberries
- 1/2 cup Greek yogurt
- 1/4 cup granola
- 1 tablespoon honey

Instructions:

- ✓ Blend bananas, blueberries, and Greek yogurt until everything is smooth.
- ✓ Transfer into bowls and top with granola and honey.

Mushroom and Spinach Frittata

Servings: 4 | Prep Time: 10 mins | Cooking Time: 20 mins

Ingredients:

- 6 large eggs
- 1 cup sliced mushrooms
- 1 cup fresh spinach

- 1/2 cup shredded Parmesan cheese
- Salt and pepper to taste

Instructions:

- ✓ Set the temperature of the oven to 350 degrees Fahrenheit (175 degrees Celsius).
- ✓ In an oven-safe skillet, sauté mushrooms and spinach until wilted.
- ✓ Whisk eggs with salt, pepper, and Parmesan cheese. Pour over veggies.
- ✓ Bake in the oven for fifteen to twenty minutes until set.

Chia Seed Pudding

Servings: 2 | Prep Time: 5 mins | Cooking Time: 0 mins

Ingredients:

- 1/4 cup chia seeds
- 1 cup almond milk
- 1 teaspoon vanilla extract
- 1 tablespoon maple syrup
- Sliced strawberries for topping

Instructions:

- ✓ In a jar, put together chia seeds, almond milk, vanilla extract, and maple syrup.
- ✓ Stir very well and refrigerate overnight.
- ✓ Top with sliced strawberries before serving.

Sweet Potato and Black Bean Breakfast Burrito

Servings: 4 | Prep Time: 15 mins | Cooking Time: 20 mins

Ingredients:

- 4 large eggs
- 1 sweet potato, diced and roasted
- 1/2 cup black beans
- 1/2 cup shredded cheddar cheese
- 4 whole-grain tortillas
- Salsa (optional)

Instructions:

- ✓ Scramble eggs in a pan, then set aside.
- ✓ Fill tortillas with eggs, sweet potatoes, black beans, and cheese.
- ✓ Roll them up and heat in a pan until the cheese melts.
- ✓ Serve with salsa if desired.

Apple Cinnamon Oatmeal

Servings: 2 | Prep Time: 5 mins | Cooking Time: 10 mins

Ingredients:

- 1 cup rolled oats
- 2 cups milk (of your choice)
- 1 apple, diced
- 1 teaspoon cinnamon
- 1 tablespoon maple syrup
- Chopped walnuts (optional)

Instructions:

- ✓ In a saucepan, put together the oats and milk. Cook over moderate to high heat until creamy.
- ✓ Stir in diced apples, cinnamon, and maple syrup.
- ✓ Top with chopped walnuts if desired.

Veggie and Cheese Breakfast Wrap

Servings: 4 | Prep Time: 10 mins | Cooking Time: 10 mins

Ingredients:

- 4 large eggs

- 1/2 cup diced bell peppers
- 1/4 cup diced tomatoes
- 1/4 cup chopped spinach
- 1/4 cup shredded mozzarella cheese
- 4 whole-grain tortillas

Instructions:

- ✓ Whisk eggs in a bowl and adjust with a little salt and pepper.
- ✓ Transfer eggs into a hot, greased pan.
- ✓ Add peppers, tomatoes, spinach, and cheese.
- ✓ Once the omelet sets, roll it in a tortilla.

Berry and Spinach Breakfast Smoothie

Servings: 2 | Prep Time: 5 mins | Cooking Time: 0 mins

Ingredients:

- 1 cup fresh spinach leaves
- 1 cup mixed berries
- 1/2 banana
- 1 cup Greek yogurt
- 1/2 cup almond milk
- 1 tablespoon honey

Instructions:

- ✓ Blend spinach, berries, banana, Greek yogurt, almond milk, and honey until everything is smooth.
- ✓ Serve chilled.

Smashed Avocado and Egg Toast

Servings: 2 | Prep Time: 10 mins | Cooking Time: 10 mins

Ingredients:

- 2 slices of whole-grain bread
- 2 ripe avocados
- 2 eggs
- Salt and pepper to taste
- Red pepper flakes (optional)

Instructions:

- ✓ Toast the bread until golden brown.
- ✓ Mash the avocado on the toast and sprinkle with a little salt and pepper.
- ✓ Fry or poach the eggs and place them on top.
- ✓ Add red pepper flakes if desired.

Mediterranean Breakfast Plate

Servings: 2 | Prep Time: 10 mins | Cooking Time: 0 mins

Ingredients:

- 2 boiled eggs
- 1/2 cup hummus
- Cherry tomatoes
- Cucumber slices
- Olives
- Feta cheese
- Whole-grain pita bread

Instructions:

- ✓ Arrange boiled eggs, hummus, cherry tomatoes, cucumber, olives, and feta cheese on a plate.
- ✓ Serve with whole-grain pita bread.

Peanut Butter and Jelly Overnight Oats

Servings: 2 | Prep Time: 5 mins | Cooking Time: 10 mins

Ingredients:

- 1 cup rolled oats

- 2 cups milk (of your choice)
- 2 tablespoons peanut butter
- 2 tablespoons jelly (your choice of flavor)
- Sliced strawberries for topping

Instructions:

- ✓ In a jar, put together the oats and milk. Stir well.
- ✓ Swirl in peanut butter and jelly.
- ✓ Refrigerate overnight and top with sliced strawberries before serving.

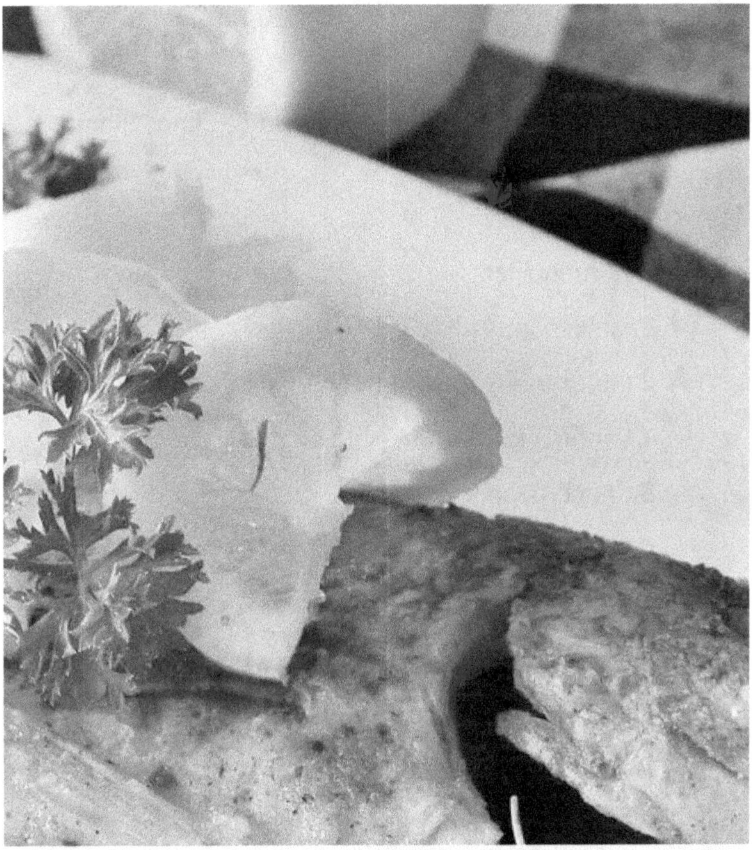

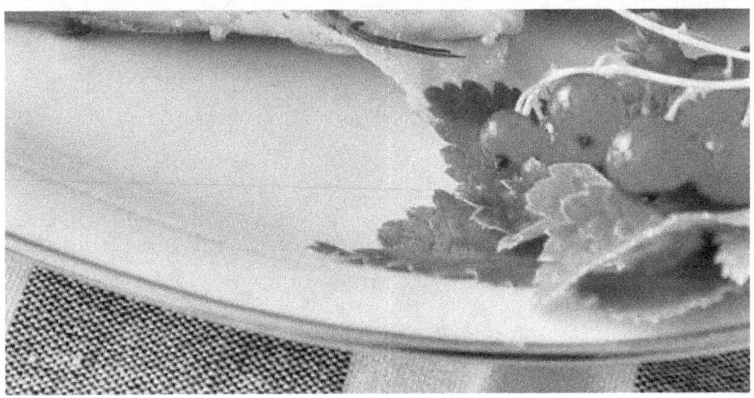

FISH AND SEAFOOD RECIPES

Baked Salmon with Dill

Servings: 2 | Prep Time: 5 mins | Cooking Time: 20 mins

Ingredients:

- 2 salmon filets
- 2 tablespoons olive oil
- 2 tablespoons fresh dill, chopped
- 1 lemon, sliced
- Salt and pepper to taste

Instructions:

- ✓ Set the temperature of the oven to 375 degrees Fahrenheit (190 degrees Celsius).
- ✓ Gently put the salmon filets on a baking sheet.
- ✓ Drizzle with olive oil, sprinkle with dill, and adjust with a little salt and pepper.
- ✓ Top with lemon slices and bake for fifteen to twenty minutes.

Lemon Garlic Shrimp Pasta

Servings: 2 | Prep Time: 10 mins | Cooking Time: 15 mins

Ingredients:

- 8 oz whole wheat pasta
- 1 lb. large shrimp, peeled and deveined
- 2 tablespoons olive oil
- 3 cloves garlic, minced
- Zest and juice of 1 lemon
- Fresh parsley for garnish
- Salt and pepper to taste

Instructions:

- ✓ Cook pasta in accordance with the package instructions.
- ✓ In a skillet, heat olive oil and sauté garlic.
- ✓ Add shrimp, lemon zest, and lemon juice. Cook until the shrimp turn pink.
- ✓ Toss cooked pasta with the shrimp mixture. Garnish with fresh parsley.

Tuna and White Bean Salad

Servings: 4 | Prep Time: 10 mins | Cooking Time: 0 mins

Ingredients:

- 2 cans (5 oz each) tuna carefully drained
- 1 can (15 oz) white beans, carefully washed and drained
- 1/4 cup red onion, finely chopped
- 1/4 cup fresh parsley, chopped
- 2 tablespoons olive oil
- 2 tablespoons red wine vinegar
- Salt and pepper to taste

Instructions:

- ✓ In a large bowl, put together tuna, white beans, red onion, and parsley.
- ✓ Sprinkle with red wine vinegar and olive oil.
- ✓ Add a little salt and pepper and toss to combine.

Grilled Lemon Herb Tilapia

Servings: 4 | Prep Time: 10 mins | Cooking Time: 10 mins

Ingredients:

- 4 tilapia filets
- 2 tablespoons olive oil
- Zest and juice of 1 lemon
- 1 teaspoon dried oregano
- 1 teaspoon dried thyme
- Salt and pepper to taste

Instructions:

- ✓ Preheat the grill to moderate to high heat.
- ✓ In a bowl, mix olive oil, lemon zest, lemon juice, oregano, thyme, salt, and pepper.
- ✓ Brush the mixture onto the tilapia filets.
- ✓ Grill for about three to four minutes per side until fish flakes easily.

Spicy Shrimp Tacos

Servings: 4 | Prep Time: 4 mins | Cooking Time: 10 mins

Ingredients:

- 1 lb large shrimp, peeled and deveined
- 1 tablespoon olive oil
- 1 teaspoon chili powder
- 1/2 teaspoon paprika
- 1/2 teaspoon cayenne pepper
- 8 small corn tortillas
- Shredded cabbage
- Sliced avocado
- Lime wedges

Instructions:

- ✓ In a bowl, toss shrimp with olive oil and spices.
- ✓ Heat a skillet and cook shrimp for two to three minutes per side.
- ✓ Serve in warm corn tortillas with shredded cabbage, avocado, and lime wedges.

Baked Cod with Tomato and Olive Salsa

Servings: 4 | Prep Time: 10 mins | Cooking Time: 20 mins

Ingredients:

- 4 cod filets
- 2 tablespoons olive oil
- 1 cup cherry tomatoes, halved
- 1/4 cup Kalamata olives, neatly pitted and chopped
- 2 cloves garlic, minced
- Fresh basil for garnish
- Salt and pepper to taste

Instructions:

- ✓ Set the temperature of the oven to 375 degrees Fahrenheit (190 degrees Celsius).
- ✓ Put the cod filets on a baking sheet.
- ✓ In a bowl, mix olive oil, cherry tomatoes, olives, garlic, salt, and pepper.
- ✓ Spoon the salsa over the fish and bake for fifteen to twenty minutes.
- ✓ Garnish with fresh basil.

Cajun Grilled Shrimp Salad

Servings: 4 | Prep Time: 10 mins | Cooking Time: 10 mins

Ingredients:

- 1 lb. large shrimp, peeled and deveined
- 2 teaspoons Cajun seasoning
- 8 cups mixed greens
- 1 red bell pepper, sliced
- 1 cucumber, sliced
- 1/4 cup red onion, thinly sliced
- 1/4 cup balsamic vinaigrette

Instructions:

1. Toss shrimp with Cajun seasoning and grill for two to three minutes per side.

2. In a large bowl, put together the mixed greens, red bell pepper, cucumber, and red onion.

3. Drizzle with balsamic vinaigrette and top with grilled shrimp.

Pesto and Tomato Baked Salmon

Servings: 2 | Prep Time: 10 mins | Cooking Time: 20 mins

Ingredients:

- 2 salmon filets
- 2 tablespoons pesto sauce
- 1 cup cherry tomatoes, halved
- 1/4 cup fresh basil, chopped
- Salt and pepper to taste

Instructions:

- ✓ Set the temperature of the oven to 375 degrees Fahrenheit (190 degrees Celsius).
- ✓ Gently put the salmon filets on a baking sheet.
- ✓ Spread pesto over the salmon, then top with cherry tomatoes and basil.
- ✓ Adjust with a little salt and pepper.
- ✓ Bake for fifteen to twenty minutes.

Coconut Lime Shrimp

Servings: 4 | Prep Time: 10 mins | Cooking Time: 10 mins

Ingredients:

- 1 lb. large shrimp, peeled and deveined
- 2 tablespoons coconut oil
- Zest and juice of 2 limes
- 1 teaspoon red pepper flakes
- Fresh cilantro for garnish
- Salt and pepper to taste

Instructions:

- ✓ In a skillet, heat coconut oil and sauté shrimp until pink.
- ✓ Add lime zest, lime juice, red pepper flakes, salt, and pepper.
- ✓ Garnish with fresh cilantro.

Tuna Stuffed Bell Peppers

Servings: 4 | Prep Time: 15 mins | Cooking Time: 25 mins

Ingredients:

- 4 bell peppers, halved with seeds carefully removed
- 2 cans (5 oz each) tuna, carefully drained
- 1/2 cup cooked quinoa
- 1/4 cup diced tomatoes
- 1/4 cup chopped parsley
- 1/4 cup feta cheese
- Salt and pepper to taste

Instructions:

- ✓ Set the temperature of the oven to 375 degrees Fahrenheit (190 degrees Celsius).
- ✓ In a bowl, put together the tuna, quinoa, tomatoes, parsley, and feta cheese.
- ✓ Adjust with a little salt and pepper.
- ✓ Stuff the bell pepper halves with the mixture and bake for twenty to twenty-five minutes.

Lemon Herb Grilled Swordfish

Servings: 4 | Prep Time: 10 mins | Cooking Time: 10 mins

Ingredients:

- 4 swordfish steaks
- 2 tablespoons olive oil
- Zest and juice of 1 lemon
- 1 teaspoon dried rosemary
- 1 teaspoon dried thyme
- Salt and pepper to taste

Instructions:

- ✓ Set the temperature of the grill to moderate to high heat.
- ✓ In a bowl, put together the olive oil, lemon zest, lemon juice, rosemary, thyme, salt, and pepper.
- ✓ Brush the mixture onto swordfish steaks.
- ✓ Grill for about three to four minutes per side until the fish is opaque.

Shrimp and Vegetable Stir-Fry

Servings: 4 | Prep Time: 10 mins | Cooking Time: 15 mins

Ingredients:

- 1 lb. large shrimp, peeled and deveined
- 2 tablespoons soy sauce
- 1 tablespoon hoisin sauce
- 1 tablespoon sesame oil
- 2 cups broccoli florets
- 1 red bell pepper, sliced
- 1 carrot, julienned
- Cooked brown rice for serving

Instructions:

- ✓ In a bowl, whisk together soy sauce, hoisin sauce, and sesame oil.
- ✓ In a wok or skillet, stir-fry shrimp and vegetables until cooked.
- ✓ Transfer the sauce over the stir-fry and serve over brown rice.

Panko-Crusted Cod with Mango Salsa

Servings: 4 | Prep Time: 10 mins | Cooking Time: 20 mins

Ingredients:

- 4 cod filets
- 1/2 cup panko breadcrumbs
- 1 teaspoon paprika
- 2 eggs, beaten
- 2 cups diced mango
- 1/4 cup red onion, finely chopped
- 1/4 cup fresh cilantro, chopped
- Lime wedges

Instructions:

- ✓ Set the temperature of the oven to 375 degrees Fahrenheit (190 degrees Celsius).
- ✓ In a bowl, put together the panko breadcrumbs and paprika.
- ✓ Dip cod filets in beaten eggs, then coat with breadcrumb mixture.
- ✓ Bake for fifteen to twenty minutes.
- ✓ In another bowl, put together the mango, red onion, and cilantro.
- ✓ Serve the cod with mango salsa and lime wedges.

Lemon Dill Shrimp Skewers

Servings: 4 | Prep Time: 10 mins | Cooking Time: 6 mins

Ingredients:

- 1 lb. large shrimp, peeled and deveined
- 2 tablespoons olive oil
- Zest and juice of 1 lemon
- 2 cloves garlic, minced
- 1 tablespoon fresh dill, chopped
- Salt and pepper to taste

Instructions:

- ✓ Preheat the grill to moderate to high temperature.
- ✓ In a bowl, put together the olive oil, lemon zest, lemon juice, garlic, dill, salt, and pepper.
- ✓ Thread shrimp on skewers and brush with the mixture.
- ✓ Grill for about two to three minutes per side until shrimp turn pink.

Teriyaki Salmon Bowl

Servings: 2 | Prep Time: 15 mins | Cooking Time: 15 mins

Ingredients:

- 2 salmon filets

- 1/4 cup teriyaki sauce

- 2 cups cooked brown rice

- 1 cup steamed broccoli

- 1/2 cup shredded carrots

- 1/4 cup sliced green onions

- Sesame seeds for garnish

Instructions:

1. Marinate salmon in teriyaki sauce for ten minutes.

2. Grill or bake the salmon until it flakes easily.

3. Assemble bowls with brown rice, salmon, broccoli, carrots, and green onions.

4. Sprinkle with sesame seeds.

Blackened Tilapia Tacos

Servings: 4 | Prep Time: 10 mins | Cooking Time: 10 mins

Ingredients:

- 4 tilapia filets
- 2 tablespoons blackened seasoning
- 8 small corn tortillas
- Shredded lettuce
- Diced tomatoes
- Sliced avocado
- Lime wedges

Instructions:

- ✓ Rub tilapia filets with blackened seasoning.
- ✓ Grill or pan-sear for two to three minutes per side until the fish is opaque.
- ✓ Serve in warm corn tortillas with lettuce, tomatoes, avocado, and lime wedges.

Shrimp and Asparagus Stir-Fry

Servings: 4 | Prep Time: 10 mins | Cooking Time: 10 mins

Ingredients:

- 1 lb. large shrimp, peeled and deveined
- 2 tablespoons olive oil
- 1 bunch asparagus, carefully trimmed and cut into 2-inch pieces
- 2 cloves garlic, minced
- 2 tablespoons soy sauce
- 1 tablespoon honey

Instructions:

- ✓ In a wok or skillet, heat olive oil and stir-fry shrimp for two to three minutes.
- ✓ Add asparagus and garlic, stir-fry for another two to three minutes.
- ✓ Stir in soy sauce and honey.
- ✓ Serve hot.

Mango Habanero Glazed Salmon

Servings: 2 | Prep Time: 10 mins | Cooking Time: 20 mins

Ingredients:

- 2 salmon filets
- 1/4 cup mango habanero sauce
- 1 lime, sliced
- Fresh cilantro for garnish
- Salt and pepper to taste

Instructions:

- ✓ Set the temperature of the oven to 375 degrees Fahrenheit (190 degrees Celsius).
- ✓ Gently transfer the salmon filets on a baking sheet.
- ✓ Brush with mango habanero sauce and adjust with a little salt and pepper.
- ✓ Top with lime slices and bake for fifteen to twenty minutes.
- ✓ Garnish with fresh cilantro.

Coconut Lime Rice with Shrimp

Servings: 4 | Prep Time: 10 mins | Cooking Time: 20 mins

Ingredients:

- 1 cup jasmine rice
- 1 3/4 cups coconut milk
- Zest and juice of 1 lime
- 1 lb. large shrimp, peeled and deveined
- 2 tablespoons coconut oil
- Salt and pepper to taste
- Fresh cilantro for garnish

Instructions:

- ✓ In a saucepan, put together the rice and coconut milk. Cook until rice is tender.
- ✓ Stir in lime zest and juice. Add a little salt and pepper.
- ✓ In a skillet, heat coconut oil and sauté shrimp until pink.
- ✓ Serve shrimp over coconut lime rice and garnish with fresh cilantro.

Lemon Garlic Butter Shrimp

Servings: 4 | Prep Time: 10 mins | Cooking Time: 10 mins

Ingredients:

- 1 lb. large shrimp, peeled and deveined
- 2 tablespoons olive oil
- 2 cloves garlic, minced
- Zest and juice of 1 lemon
- 2 tablespoons butter
- Fresh parsley for garnish
- Salt and pepper to taste

Instructions:

- ✓ In a skillet, heat olive oil and sauté shrimp for two to three minutes per side.
- ✓ Add garlic, lemon zest, lemon juice, butter, salt, and pepper.
- ✓ Cook for an additional two minutes.
- ✓ Garnish with fresh parsley.

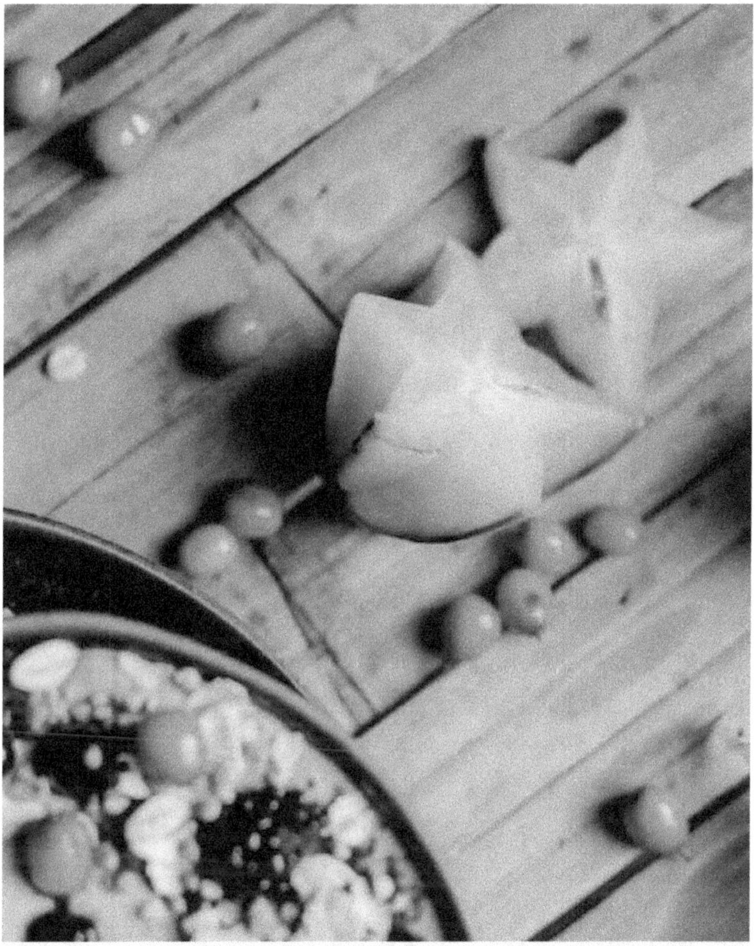

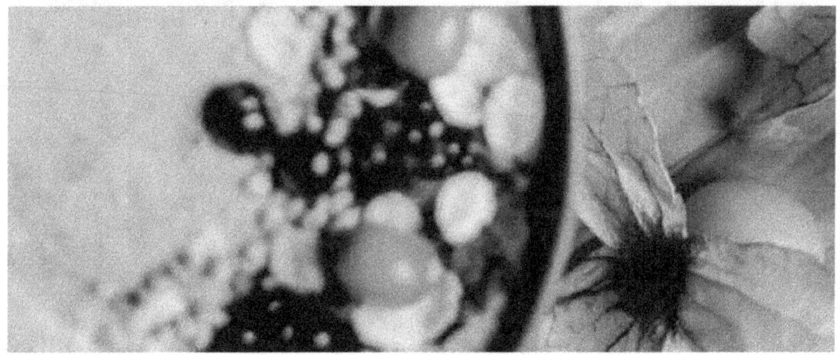
BEANS, GRAINS, AND PASTA

Quinoa and Black Bean Stuffed Peppers

Servings: 4 | Prep Time: 15 mins | Cooking Time: 30 mins

Ingredients:

- 4 bell peppers, halved with seeds carefully removed
- 1 cup cooked quinoa
- 1 can (15 oz) black beans, carefully washed and drained
- 1 cup corn kernels
- 1 cup salsa
- 1 cup shredded cheddar cheese
- Fresh cilantro for garnish

Instructions:

- ✓ Set the temperature of the oven to 375 degrees Fahrenheit (190 degrees Celsius).
- ✓ In a bowl, put together the quinoa, black beans, corn, and salsa.
- ✓ Fill bell pepper halves with the mixture and place in a baking dish.
- ✓ Top with cheddar cheese.
- ✓ Bake for twenty-five to thirty minutes or until peppers are tender.
- ✓ Garnish with fresh cilantro.

Mediterranean Chickpea Salad

Servings: 4 | Prep Time: 15 mins | Cooking Time: 0 mins

Ingredients:

- 2 cans (15 oz each) chickpeas, carefully washed and drained
- 1 cucumber, diced
- 1 red bell pepper, diced
- 1/4 cup red onion, finely chopped
- 1/4 cup Kalamata olives, pitted and finely chopped
- 1/4 cup feta cheese, crumbled
- Fresh parsley for garnish
- Greek vinaigrette dressing

Instructions:

- ✓ In a large bowl, put together the chickpeas, cucumber, red bell pepper, red onion, and olives.
- ✓ Drizzle with Greek vinaigrette dressing.
- ✓ Top with feta cheese and garnish with fresh parsley.

Lemon Garlic Shrimp and Broccoli Pasta

Servings: 2 | Prep Time: 15 mins | Cooking Time: 15 mins

Ingredients:

- 8 oz whole wheat pasta
- 1 lb. large shrimp, peeled and veins removed
- 2 tablespoons olive oil
- 3 cloves garlic, minced
- Zest and juice of 1 lemon
- 2 cups broccoli florets
- Fresh parsley for garnish
- Salt and pepper to taste

Instructions:

- ✓ Cook pasta in accordance with the package instructions.
- ✓ In a skillet, heat olive oil and sauté shrimp for two to three minutes.
- ✓ Add garlic, lemon zest, lemon juice, and broccoli. Cook until the broccoli is tender.
- ✓ Toss cooked pasta with the shrimp mixture.
- ✓ Garnish with fresh parsley.

Black Bean and Corn Quesadillas

Servings: 4 | Prep Time: 10 mins | Cooking Time: 10 mins

Ingredients:

- 4 whole-grain tortillas
- 1 can (15 oz) black beans, carefully washed and drained
- 1 cup corn kernels
- 1/2 cup shredded cheddar cheese
- 1/4 cup diced red onion
- Salsa and Greek yogurt for dipping

Instructions:

- ✓ In a bowl, put together the black beans, corn, and red onion.
- ✓ Place a tortilla in a hot, greased skillet.
- ✓ Sprinkle with cheese and add a quarter of the bean mixture.
- ✓ Top with another tortilla and press down gently.
- ✓ Cook for two to three minutes per side or until golden and cheese melts.
- ✓ Cut into wedges and serve with salsa and Greek yogurt for dipping.

Pesto and Sun-Dried Tomato Pasta

Servings: 2 | Prep Time: 10 mins | Cooking Time: 10 mins

Ingredients:

- 8 oz whole wheat pasta
- 1/2 cup sun-dried tomatoes, chopped
- 1/4 cup pesto sauce
- 1/4 cup grated Parmesan cheese
- Fresh basil for garnish
- Salt and pepper to taste

Instructions:

- ✓ Cook pasta in accordance with the package instructions.
- ✓ In a bowl, toss cooked pasta with sun-dried tomatoes, pesto sauce, and Parmesan cheese.
- ✓ Adjust with a little salt and pepper to your preferred taste.
- ✓ Garnish with fresh basil.

Spicy Black Bean and Quinoa Bowl

Servings: 2 | Prep Time: 10 mins | Cooking Time: 0 mins

Ingredients:

- 1 cup cooked quinoa
- 1 can (15 oz) black beans, carefully washed and drained
- 1 cup corn kernels
- 1 avocado, sliced
- 1/4 cup diced red onion
- Salsa and Greek yogurt for topping

Instructions:

- ✓ In a bowl, put together the cooked quinoa, black beans, corn, avocado, and red onion.
- ✓ Top with salsa and a dollop of Greek yogurt.

Lemon Garlic White Bean Salad

Servings: 4 | Prep Time: 10 mins | Cooking Time: 0 mins

Ingredients:

- 2 cans (15 oz each) white beans, washed and drained
- 1/4 cup fresh parsley, chopped

- 2 cloves garlic, minced
- Zest and juice of 1 lemon
- 2 tablespoons olive oil
- Salt and pepper to taste

Instructions:

- ✓ In a bowl, put together the white beans, parsley, garlic, lemon zest, lemon juice, and olive oil.
- ✓ Add a little salt and pepper to your preferred taste.
- ✓ Chill before serving.

Mediterranean Orzo Salad

Servings: 4 | Prep Time: 10 mins | Cooking Time: 10 mins

Ingredients:

- 1 cup whole wheat orzo
- 1/2 cup cherry tomatoes, halved
- 1/4 cup Kalamata olives, pitted and finely chopped
- 1/4 cup feta cheese, crumbled
- 1/4 cup fresh parsley, chopped
- Lemon vinaigrette dressing

Instructions:

- ✓ Cook orzo in accordance with package instructions.

- ✓ In a bowl, put together the orzo, cherry tomatoes, olives, feta cheese, and parsley.
- ✓ Drizzle with lemon vinaigrette dressing.

Black Bean and Sweet Potato Tacos

Servings: 4 | Prep Time: 10 mins | Cooking Time: 10 mins

Ingredients:

- 8 small whole-grain tortillas
- 1 can (15 oz) black beans, carefully washed and drained
- 2 cups sweet potatoes, finely peeled and diced
- 1 teaspoon chili powder
- 1/2 teaspoon cumin
- Salsa and Greek yogurt for topping

Instructions:

- ✓ In a skillet, sauté sweet potatoes with chili powder and cumin until tender.
- ✓ Add black beans and cook for an additional two to three minutes.
- ✓ Heat tortillas and fill with the sweet potato and black bean mixture.

✓ Top with salsa and a dollop of Greek yogurt.

Avocado and Chickpea Salad

Servings: 4 | Prep Time: 10 mins | Cooking Time: 0 mins

Ingredients:

- 2 cans (15 oz each) chickpeas, carefully washed and drained
- 2 ripe avocados, diced
- 1/4 cup red onion, finely chopped
- 1/4 cup fresh cilantro, chopped
- 2 tablespoons olive oil
- 2 tablespoons lemon juice
- Salt and pepper to taste

Instructions:

✓ In a bowl, put together the chickpeas, avocados, red onion, and cilantro.

✓ Splash with lemon juice and olive oil.

✓ Adjust with a little salt and pepper to your preferred taste.

Lemon Garlic Quinoa with Spinach

Servings: 2 | Prep Time: 10 mins | Cooking Time: 10 mins

Ingredients:

- 1 cup cooked quinoa
- 2 cups fresh spinach
- 2 cloves garlic, minced
- Zest and juice of 1 lemon
- 2 tablespoons olive oil
- Salt and pepper to taste

Instructions:

- ✓ In a skillet, sauté garlic in olive oil until fragrant.
- ✓ Add fresh spinach and cook until wilted.
- ✓ Stir in cooked quinoa, lemon zest, lemon juice, salt, and pepper.
- ✓ Toss to combine.

Tomato Basil Pasta with White Beans

Servings: 2 | Prep Time: 10 mins | Cooking Time: 10 mins

Ingredients:

- 8 oz whole wheat pasta
- 1 can (15 oz) white beans, carefully washed and drained
- 1 cup cherry tomatoes, halved
- 1/4 cup fresh basil, chopped
- 2 tablespoons olive oil
- 2 cloves garlic, minced
- Salt and pepper to taste

Instructions:

- ✓ Cook pasta in accordance with the package instructions.
- ✓ In a bowl, put together the white beans, cherry tomatoes, and fresh basil.
- ✓ In a skillet, sauté garlic in olive oil until fragrant.
- ✓ Toss cooked pasta with the white bean mixture.
- ✓ Adjust with a little salt and pepper to your preferred taste.

Caprese Quinoa Salad

Servings: 2 | Prep Time: 10 mins | Cooking Time: 0 mins

Ingredients:

- 1 cup cooked quinoa
- 1 cup cherry tomatoes, halved
- 1 cup fresh mozzarella balls, halved
- 1/4 cup fresh basil, chopped
- 2 tablespoons balsamic vinegar
- 2 tablespoons olive oil
- Salt and pepper to taste

Instructions:

- ✓ In a bowl, put together the quinoa, cherry tomatoes, mozzarella balls, and fresh basil.
- ✓ Drizzle with balsamic vinegar and olive oil.
- ✓ Adjust with a little salt and pepper to your preferred taste.

Butternut Squash and Black Bean Enchiladas

Servings: 4 | Prep Time: 15 mins | Cooking Time: 20 mins

Ingredients:

- 8 whole-grain tortillas
- 2 cups butternut squash, diced and roasted
- 1 can (15 oz) black beans, carefully washed and drained
- 1/2 cup diced red onion
- 1/2 cup shredded cheddar cheese
- Salsa and Greek yogurt for topping

Instructions:

- ✓ Fill tortillas with roasted butternut squash, black beans, red onion, and cheddar cheese.
- ✓ Roll them up and place in a baking dish.
- ✓ Bake at 375 degrees Fahrenheit (190 degrees Celsius) for fifteen to twenty minutes.
- ✓ Serve with salsa and a dollop of Greek yogurt.

Lemon Herb Couscous with Chickpeas

Servings: 2 | Prep Time: 10 mins | Cooking Time: 10 mins

Ingredients:

- 1 cup couscous
- 2 cups vegetable broth
- 1 can (15 oz) chickpeas, carefully washed and drained
- Zest and juice of 1 lemon
- 2 tablespoons fresh parsley, chopped
- Salt and pepper to taste

Instructions:

- ✓ In a saucepan, bring vegetable broth to a boil.
- ✓ Stir in couscous, remove from heat, and cover. Let sit for five minutes.
- ✓ Fluff couscous with a fork and add chickpeas, lemon zest, lemon juice, parsley, salt, and pepper.

Spinach and White Bean Stuffed Mushrooms

Servings: 4 | Prep Time: 15 mins | Cooking Time: 25 mins

Ingredients:

- 12 large mushrooms, stems removed
- 1 can (15 oz) white beans, carefully washed and drained
- 1 cup fresh spinach, chopped
- 1/4 cup grated Parmesan cheese
- 2 cloves garlic, minced
- 2 tablespoons olive oil
- Salt and pepper to taste

Instructions:

- ✓ Set the temperature of the oven to 375 degrees Fahrenheit (190 degrees Celsius).
- ✓ In a skillet, heat olive oil and sauté garlic until fragrant.
- ✓ Add chopped spinach and cook until wilted.
- ✓ In a bowl, put together the mashed white beans, sautéed spinach, and grated Parmesan cheese.
- ✓ Stuff mushroom caps with the mixture and bake for twenty to twenty-five minutes.

Sweet Potato and Black Bean Bowl

Servings: 4 | Prep Time: 10 mins | Cooking Time: 0 mins

Ingredients:

- 2 cups cooked sweet potatoes, diced
- 1 can (15 oz) black beans, carefully washed and drained
- 1 cup corn kernels (fresh or frozen)
- 1/4 cup diced red onion
- 1/4 cup fresh cilantro, chopped
- Lime wedges

Instructions:

- ✓ In a bowl, put together the cooked sweet potatoes, black beans, corn, red onion, and cilantro.
- ✓ Squeeze fresh lime juice over the top before serving.

Lemon Garlic White Bean Dip

Servings: 4 | Prep Time: 10 mins | Cooking Time: 0 mins

Ingredients:

- 1 can (15 oz) white beans, carefully washed and drained
- 2 cloves garlic, minced
- Zest and juice of 1 lemon
- 2 tablespoons olive oil
- Fresh parsley for garnish
- Salt and pepper to taste

Instructions:

- ✓ In a food processor, put together the white beans, garlic, lemon zest, lemon juice, and olive oil.
- ✓ Blend until everything is smooth.
- ✓ Adjust with a little salt and pepper to your preferred taste.
- ✓ Garnish with fresh parsley.

Mediterranean Lentil Salad

Servings: 2 | Prep Time: 10 mins | Cooking Time: 0 mins

Ingredients:

- 1 cup cooked brown lentils
- 1/2 cup cherry tomatoes, halved
- 1/4 cup Kalamata olives, pitted and chopped
- 1/4 cup crumbled feta cheese

- 2 tablespoons olive oil
- 2 tablespoons balsamic vinegar
- Fresh parsley for garnish
- Salt and pepper to taste

Instructions:

- ✓ In a bowl, combine cooked brown lentils, cherry tomatoes, Kalamata olives, and feta cheese.
- ✓ Drizzle with olive oil and balsamic vinegar.
- ✓ Add a little salt and pepper to your preferred taste.
- ✓ Garnish with fresh parsley.

Quinoa and White Bean Stuffed Bell Peppers

Servings: 4 | Prep Time: 15 mins | Cooking Time: 25 mins

Ingredients:

- 4 bell peppers, halved with seeds removed
- 1 cup cooked quinoa
- 1 can (15 oz) white beans, carefully washed and drained
- 1/4 cup diced tomatoes
- 1/4 cup fresh basil, chopped
- 1/4 cup feta cheese

🌶 Salt and pepper to taste

Instructions:

- ✓ Set the temperature of the oven to 375 degrees Fahrenheit (190 degrees Celsius).
- ✓ In a bowl, put together the cooked quinoa, white beans, diced tomatoes, basil, and feta cheese.
- ✓ Adjust with a little salt and pepper to your preferred taste.
- ✓ Stuff bell pepper halves with the mixture and bake for twenty to twenty-five minutes.

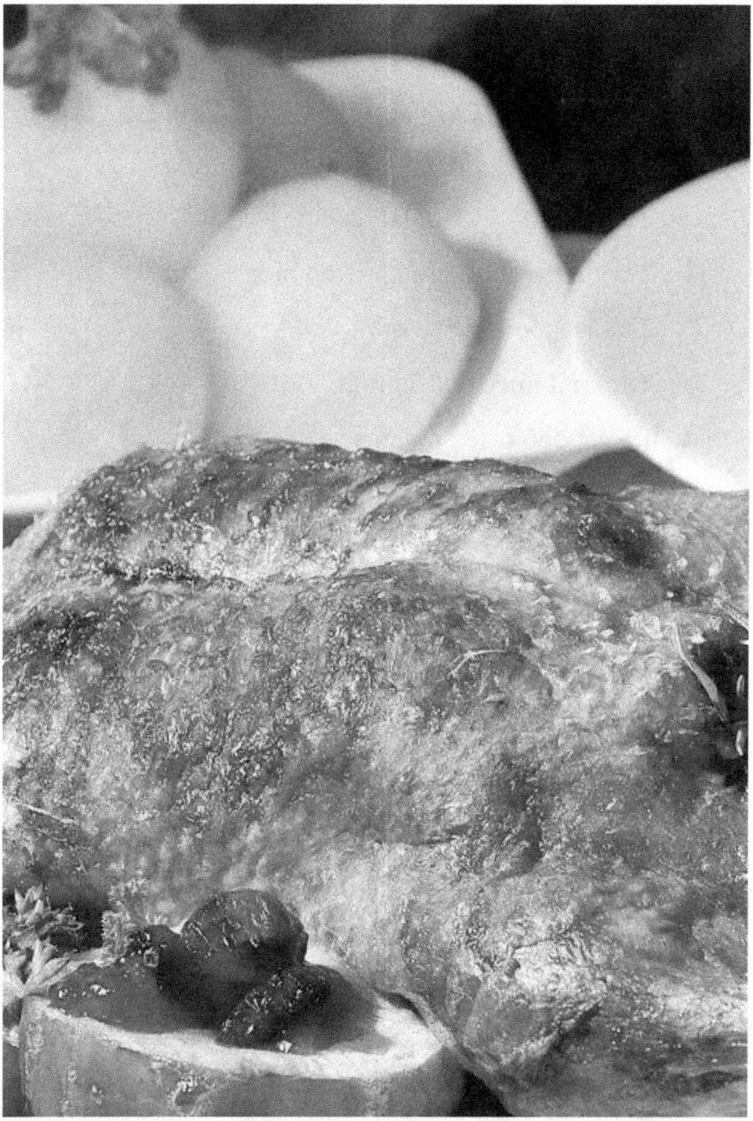

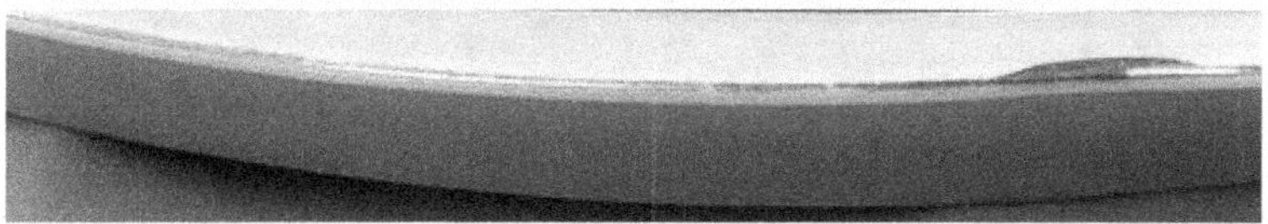

POULTRY AND MEAT RECIPES

Lemon Herb Grilled Chicken

Servings: 2 | Prep Time: 10 mins | Cooking Time: 16 mins

Ingredients:

- 2 boneless, skinless chicken breasts
- 2 tablespoons olive oil
- Zest and juice of 1 lemon
- 1 teaspoon dried rosemary
- 1 teaspoon dried thyme
- Salt and pepper to taste

Instructions:

- ✓ Preheat the grill to moderate to high temperature.
- ✓ In a bowl, mix olive oil, lemon zest, lemon juice, rosemary, thyme, salt, and pepper.
- ✓ Brush the mixture onto chicken breasts.
- ✓ Grill for about six to eight minutes per side until chicken is no longer pink in the center.

Balsamic Glazed Turkey Breast

Servings: 2 | Prep Time: 15 mins | Cooking Time: 10 mins

Ingredients:

- 2 turkey breast cutlets
- 1/4 cup balsamic vinegar
- 2 tablespoons honey
- 2 cloves garlic, minced
- 1 teaspoon dried thyme
- Salt and pepper to taste

Instructions:

- ✓ In a bowl, whisk together balsamic vinegar, honey, garlic, thyme, salt, and pepper.
- ✓ Marinate turkey cutlets in the mixture for fifteen minutes.
- ✓ Heat a skillet over moderate to high heat and cook turkey for three to four minutes per side until no longer pink.

Mediterranean Chicken and Vegetable Skewers

Servings: 2 | Prep Time: 15 mins | Cooking Time: 10 mins

Ingredients:

- 2 boneless, skinless chicken breasts, which is cut into cubes
- 1 zucchini, sliced into rounds
- 1 red bell pepper, cut into chunks
- 1 red onion, cut into wedges
- 2 tablespoons olive oil
- 1 teaspoon dried oregano
- Salt and pepper to taste

Instructions:

- ✓ Thread chicken and vegetables onto skewers.
- ✓ In a bowl, mix olive oil, oregano, salt, and pepper.
- ✓ Brush the mixture onto the skewers.
- ✓ Grill for four to five minutes per side until chicken is cooked through.

Rosemary and Garlic Roasted Chicken

Servings: 2 | Prep Time: 10 mins | Cooking Time: 35 mins

Ingredients:

- 4 bone-in, skin-on chicken thighs
- 2 tablespoons olive oil
- 3 cloves garlic, minced
- 1 teaspoon dried rosemary
- 1/2 teaspoon paprika
- Salt and pepper to taste

Instructions:

- ✓ Set the temperature of the oven to 375 degrees Fahrenheit (190 degrees Celsius).
- ✓ In a bowl, mix olive oil, garlic, rosemary, paprika, salt, and pepper.
- ✓ Rub the mixture onto chicken thighs.
- ✓ Roast for 30-35 minutes until the chicken reaches an internal temperature of 165 degrees Fahrenheit (74 degrees Celsius).

Ginger Soy Chicken Stir-Fry

Servings: 2 | Prep Time: 15 mins | Cooking Time: 15 mins

Ingredients:

- 2 boneless, skinless chicken breasts, cut into strips
- 2 tablespoons soy sauce
- 1 tablespoon fresh ginger, minced
- 2 cloves garlic, minced
- 2 cups mixed vegetables (broccoli, bell peppers, snap peas)
- 2 tablespoons sesame oil
- Cooked brown rice for serving

Instructions:

- ✓ In a bowl, marinate chicken in soy sauce, ginger, and garlic for fifteen minutes.
- ✓ In a wok or skillet, heat sesame oil and stir-fry chicken until no longer pink.
- ✓ Add mixed vegetables and continue stir-frying until tender.
- ✓ Serve over cooked brown rice.

Lemon Pepper Grilled Turkey Burgers

Servings: 4 | Prep Time: 10 mins | Cooking Time: 14 mins

Ingredients:

- 1 lb. ground turkey
- Zest and juice of 1 lemon
- 1 teaspoon black pepper
- 1/2 teaspoon garlic powder
- 4 whole-grain burger buns
- Lettuce, tomato, and red

Instructions:

- ✓ In a bowl, mix ground turkey, lemon zest, lemon juice, black pepper, and garlic powder.
- ✓ Shape into four patties.
- ✓ Preheat the grill to moderate to high heat and grill for about five to seven minutes per side.
- ✓ Serve on whole-grain buns with your choice of toppings.

Herb-Roasted Chicken Drumsticks

Servings: 4 | Prep Time: 10 mins | Cooking Time: 35 mins

Ingredients:

- 8 chicken drumsticks
- 2 tablespoons olive oil
- 1 teaspoon dried thyme
- 1 teaspoon dried rosemary
- 1/2 teaspoon paprika
- Salt and pepper to taste

Instructions:

- ✓ Set the temperature of the oven to 375 degrees Fahrenheit (190 degrees Celsius).
- ✓ In a bowl, mix olive oil, thyme, rosemary, paprika, salt, and pepper.
- ✓ Rub the mixture onto chicken drumsticks.
- ✓ Roast for thirty to thirty-five minutes until chicken is cooked through.

Teriyaki Turkey and Broccoli Stir-Fry

Servings: 4 | Prep Time: 10 mins | Cooking Time: 15 mins

Ingredients:

- 1 lb. ground turkey
- 2 tablespoons teriyaki sauce
- 2 cups broccoli florets
- 1 red bell pepper, sliced
- 2 cloves garlic, minced
- 2 tablespoons sesame oil
- Cooked brown rice for serving

Instructions:

- ✓ In a skillet, cook ground turkey until browned.
- ✓ Stir in teriyaki sauce.
- ✓ Add broccoli, red bell pepper, and garlic, and stir-fry until vegetables are tender.
- ✓ Serve over cooked brown rice.

Rosemary Balsamic Grilled Chicken

Servings: 2 | Prep Time: 15 mins | Cooking Time: 16 mins

Ingredients:

- 2 boneless, skinless chicken breasts
- 2 tablespoons balsamic vinegar
- 1 tablespoon olive oil
- 1 teaspoon dried rosemary
- 2 cloves garlic, minced
- Salt and pepper to taste

Instructions:

- ✓ In a bowl, mix balsamic vinegar, olive oil, rosemary, garlic, salt, and pepper.
- ✓ Marinate chicken breasts in the mixture for 15 minutes.
- ✓ Preheat the grill to moderate to high heat and grill for about six to seven minutes per side until the chicken is no longer pink in the center.

Mediterranean Turkey and Quinoa Bowl

Servings: 2 | Prep Time: 10 mins | Cooking Time: 10 mins

Ingredients:

- 1 cup cooked quinoa
- 1/2 lb. ground turkey
- 1/2 teaspoon dried oregano
- 1/4 cup cherry tomatoes, halved
- 1/4 cup Kalamata olives, pitted and chopped
- 1/4 cup feta cheese, crumbled
- Greek vinaigrette dressing

Instructions:

- ✓ In a skillet, cook ground turkey with dried oregano until browned.
- ✓ In a bowl, put together the cooked quinoa, turkey, cherry tomatoes, olives, and feta cheese.
- ✓ Drizzle with Greek vinaigrette dressing.

Lemon Garlic Pork Chops

Servings: 2 | Prep Time: 10 mins | Cooking Time: 10 mins

Ingredients:

- 2 boneless pork chops
- 2 tablespoons olive oil
- Zest and juice of 1 lemon
- 2 cloves garlic, minced
- 1/2 teaspoon dried thyme
- Salt and pepper to taste

Instructions:

- ✓ In a bowl, put together the olive oil, lemon zest, lemon juice, garlic, thyme, salt, and pepper.
- ✓ Brush the mixture onto pork chops.
- ✓ Heat a skillet over moderate to high heat and cook pork chops for four to five minutes per side until no longer pink in the center.

BBQ Chicken and Vegetable Skewers

Servings: 2 | Prep Time: 15 mins | Cooking Time: 10 mins

Ingredients:

- 2 boneless, skinless chicken breasts, which is cut into cubes
- 1 zucchini, sliced into rounds
- 1 red bell pepper, cut into chunks
- 1 red onion, cut into wedges
- 1/4 cup BBQ sauce
- Salt and pepper to taste

Instructions:

- ✓ Thread chicken and vegetables onto skewers.
- ✓ Brush with BBQ sauce, and adjust with a little salt and pepper.
- ✓ Grill for four to five minutes per side until chicken is cooked through.

Greek-Style Lamb and Couscous Bowl

Servings: 2 | Prep Time: 10 mins | Cooking Time: 10 mins

Ingredients:

- 1 cup cooked whole wheat couscous
- 1/2 lb. ground lamb
- 1/2 teaspoon dried oregano
- 1/4 cup cherry tomatoes, halved
- 1/4 cup Kalamata olives, pitted and chopped
- 1/4 cup crumbled feta cheese
- Tzatziki sauce for topping

Instructions:

- ✓ In a skillet, cook ground lamb with dried oregano until browned.
- ✓ In a bowl, put together the cooked couscous, lamb, cherry tomatoes, olives, and feta cheese.
- ✓ Serve with a dollop of tzatziki sauce.

Honey Mustard Grilled Chicken

Servings: 2 | Prep Time: 10 mins | Cooking Time: 16 mins

Ingredients:

- 2 boneless, skinless chicken breasts
- 1/4 cup Dijon mustard
- 2 tablespoons honey
- 1 clove garlic, minced
- Salt and pepper to taste

Instructions:

- ✓ In a bowl, put together the Dijon mustard, honey, garlic, salt, and pepper.
- ✓ Brush the mixture onto chicken breasts.
- ✓ Set the temperature of the grill to medium-high heat and grill for about six to eight minutes per side until the chicken is no longer pink in the center.

Beef and Broccoli Stir-Fry

Servings: 2 | Prep Time: 15 mins | Cooking Time: 10 mins

Ingredients:

- 1/2 lb. flank steak, thinly sliced
- 2 tablespoons soy sauce
- 1 tablespoon hoisin sauce
- 1 tablespoon sesame oil
- 2 cups broccoli florets
- 2 cloves garlic, minced
- Cooked brown rice for serving

Instructions:

- ✓ In a bowl, marinate steak in soy sauce, hoisin sauce, and sesame oil for fifteen minutes.
- ✓ In a wok or skillet, stir-fry steak and garlic for two to three minutes.
- ✓ Add broccoli and continue stir-frying until tender.
- ✓ Serve over cooked brown rice.

Lemon Garlic Herb Pork Tenderloin

Servings: 2 | Prep Time: 10 mins | Cooking Time: 30 mins

Ingredients:

- 1 pork tenderloin
- 2 tablespoons olive oil
- Zest and juice of 1 lemon
- 2 cloves garlic, minced
- 1 teaspoon dried thyme
- Salt and pepper to taste

Instructions:

- ✓ Set the temperature of the oven to 375 degrees Fahrenheit (190 degrees Celsius).
- ✓ In a bowl, put together the olive oil, lemon zest, lemon juice, garlic, thyme, salt, and pepper.
- ✓ Rub the mixture onto pork tenderloin.
- ✓ Roast for twenty-five to thirty minutes until the pork reaches an internal temperature of 145 degrees Fahrenheit (63 degrees Celsius).

Spicy BBQ Turkey Burger

Servings: 4 | Prep Time: 10 mins | Cooking Time: 14 mins

Ingredients:

- 1 lb. ground turkey
- 1/4 cup BBQ sauce
- 1 teaspoon chili powder
- 1/2 teaspoon cumin
- 4 whole-grain burger buns
- Lettuce, tomato, and red onion

Instructions:

- ✓ In a bowl, put together the ground turkey, BBQ sauce, chili powder, and cumin.
- ✓ Shape into four patties.
- ✓ Set the temperature of the grill to medium-high heat and grill for about five to seven minutes per side.
- ✓ Serve on whole-grain buns with your choice of toppings.

Italian Herb Grilled Chicken

Servings: 2 | Prep Time: 10 mins | Cooking Time: 16 mins

Ingredients:

- 2 boneless, skinless chicken breasts
- 2 tablespoons olive oil
- 1 teaspoon dried Italian seasoning
- 2 cloves garlic, minced
- Salt and pepper to taste

Instructions:

- ✓ Set the temperature of the grill to moderate to high heat.
- ✓ In a bowl, put together olive oil, Italian seasoning, garlic, salt, and pepper.
- ✓ Brush the mixture onto chicken breasts.
- ✓ Grill for about six to eight minutes per side until chicken is no longer pink in the center.

Beef and Mushroom Stuffed Bell Peppers

Servings: 4 | Prep Time: 15 mins | Cooking Time: 25 mins

Ingredients:

- 4 bell peppers, halved with seeds removed
- 1/2 lb. lean ground beef
- 1 cup mushrooms, chopped
- 1/2 cup diced tomatoes
- 1/4 cup onion, finely chopped
- 1/4 cup shredded mozzarella cheese
- Italian seasoning for seasoning
- Salt and pepper to taste

Instructions:

- ✓ Set the temperature of the oven to 375 degrees Fahrenheit (190 degrees Celsius).
- ✓ In a skillet, cook ground beef and mushrooms until browned.
- ✓ Stir in diced tomatoes, onion, Italian seasoning, salt, and pepper to your preferred taste.
- ✓ Fill bell pepper halves with the mixture and top with mozzarella cheese.
- ✓ Bake for twenty to twenty-five minutes.

Lemon Garlic Chicken and Asparagus

Servings: 2 | Prep Time: 10 mins | Cooking Time: 25 mins

Ingredients:

- 2 boneless, skinless chicken breasts
- 2 tablespoons olive oil
- Zest and juice of 1 lemon
- 2 cloves garlic, minced
- 1 bunch asparagus, trimmed
- Salt and pepper to taste

Instructions:

- ✓ Set the temperature of the oven to 375 degrees Fahrenheit (190 degrees Celsius).
- ✓ In a bowl, put together the olive oil, lemon zest, lemon juice, garlic, salt, and pepper.
- ✓ Place chicken and asparagus on a baking sheet, and drizzle with the mixture.
- ✓ Roast for twenty to twenty-five minutes until chicken is cooked through.

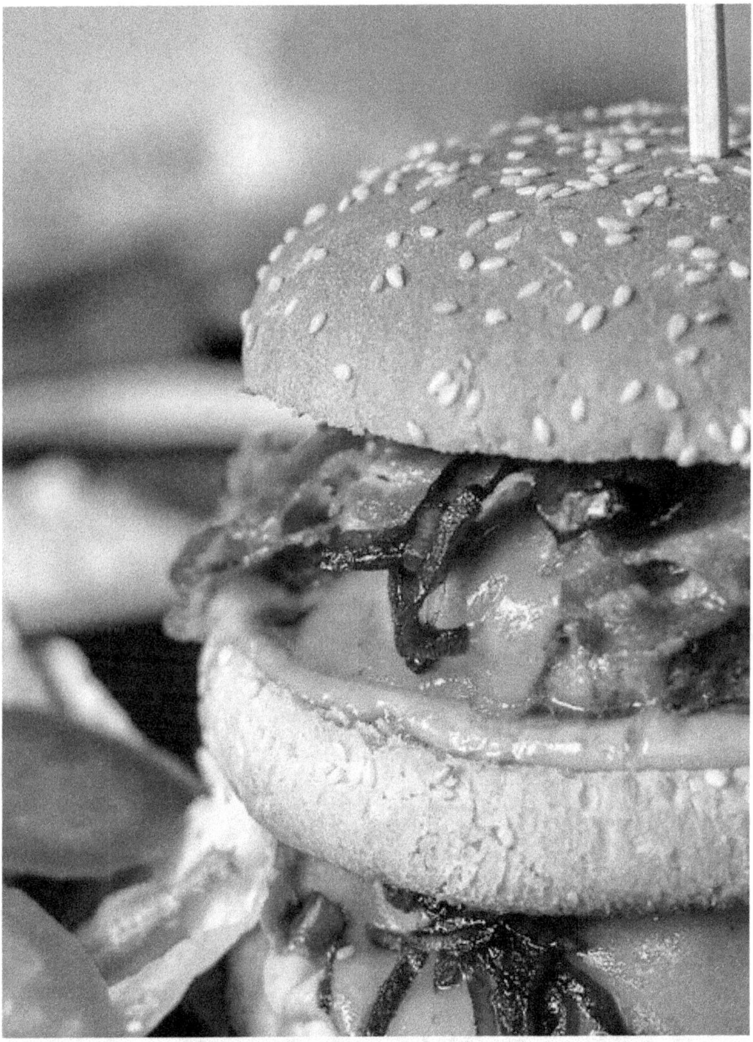

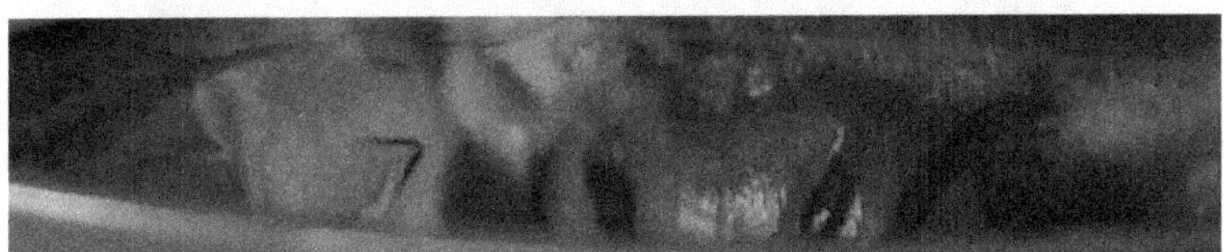

VEGAN AND VEGETARIAN RECIPES

Quinoa and Black Bean Stuffed Peppers

Servings: 4 | Prep Time: 15 mins | Cooking Time: 25 mins

Ingredients:

- 4 bell peppers, halved with seeds removed
- 1 cup cooked quinoa
- 1 can (15 oz) black beans, carefully washed and drained
- 1 cup corn kernels (fresh or frozen)
- 1/4 cup diced red onion
- 1/4 cup fresh cilantro, chopped
- Salsa for topping

Instructions:

- ✓ Set the temperature of the oven to 375 degrees Fahrenheit (190 degrees Celsius).
- ✓ In a bowl, combine the cooked quinoa, black beans, corn, red onion, and cilantro.
- ✓ Fill bell pepper halves with the mixture.
- ✓ Bake for twenty to twenty-five minutes.
- ✓ Serve with salsa on top.

Chickpea and Spinach Curry

Servings: 4 | Prep Time: 15 mins | Cooking Time: 20 mins

Ingredients:

- 2 cans (15 oz each) chickpeas, carefully washed and drained
- 2 cups fresh spinach
- 1 onion, finely chopped
- 2 cloves garlic, minced
- 1 can (15 oz) diced tomatoes
- 2 tablespoons curry powder
- 1 tablespoon olive oil
- Salt and pepper to taste

Instructions:

- ✓ In a pot, sauté onion and garlic in olive oil until fragrant.
- ✓ Stir in curry powder and cook for one minute.
- ✓ Add chickpeas, diced tomatoes, and spinach.
- ✓ Simmer for fifteen to twenty minutes, stirring occasionally.
- ✓ Adjust with a little salt and pepper to your preferred taste.

Mango and Black Bean Salad

Servings: 4 | Prep Time: 10 mins | Cooking Time: 0 mins

Ingredients:

- 1 can (15 oz) black beans, carefully washed and drained
- 2 ripe mangoes, diced
- 1 red bell pepper, diced
- 1/4 cup red onion, finely chopped
- 1/4 cup fresh cilantro, chopped
- Juice of 2 limes
- Salt and pepper to taste

Instructions:

- ✓ In a bowl, put together the black beans, diced mangoes, red bell pepper, red onion, and cilantro.
- ✓ Squeeze lime juice over the top.
- ✓ Adjust with a little salt and pepper to your preferred taste.

Sweet Potato and Chickpea Curry

Servings: 4 | Prep Time: 15 mins | Cooking Time: 25 mins

Ingredients:

- 2 sweet potatoes, peeled and diced
- 2 cans (15 oz each) chickpeas, carefully washed and drained
- 1 onion, finely chopped
- 2 cloves garlic, minced
- 1 can (15 oz) diced tomatoes
- 2 tablespoons curry powder
- 1 tablespoon olive oil
- Salt and pepper to taste

Instructions:

- ✓ In a pot, sauté onion and garlic in olive oil until fragrant.
- ✓ Stir in curry powder and cook for 1 minute.
- ✓ Add sweet potatoes, chickpeas, diced tomatoes, and enough water to cover.
- ✓ Simmer for twenty to twenty-five minutes until sweet potatoes are tender.
- ✓ Adjust with a little salt and pepper to your preferred taste.

Roasted Red Pepper and Walnut Dip

Servings: 4 | Prep Time: 15 mins | Roasting Time: 20 mins

Ingredients:

- 2 red bell peppers
- 1/2 cup walnuts, toasted
- 2 cloves garlic
- 2 tablespoons olive oil
- Juice of 1 lemon
- Salt and pepper to taste

Instructions:

- ✓ Set the temperature of the oven to 400 degrees Fahrenheit (200 degrees Celsius).
- ✓ Roast red bell peppers until skin is charred, then peel and seed them.
- ✓ In a food processor, put together the roasted red peppers, walnuts, garlic, olive oil, and lemon juice.
- ✓ Blend until everything is smooth.
- ✓ Adjust with salt and pepper to your preferred taste.

Caprese Stuffed Portobello Mushrooms

Servings: 4 | Prep Time: 15 mins | Cooking Time: 20 mins

Ingredients:

- 4 large Portobello mushrooms
- 1 cup cherry tomatoes, halved
- 1 cup fresh mozzarella balls, halved
- 1/4 cup fresh basil, chopped
- 2 tablespoons balsamic vinegar
- 2 tablespoons olive oil
- Salt and pepper to taste

Instructions:

- ✓ Set the temperature of the oven to 375 degrees Fahrenheit (190 degrees Celsius).
- ✓ Take off the stems and gills from the mushrooms.
- ✓ In a bowl, put together the cherry tomatoes, mozzarella balls, and fresh basil.
- ✓ Drizzle with balsamic vinegar and olive oil.
- ✓ Fill each mushroom cap with the mixture.
- ✓ Bake for fifteen to twenty minutes.

Chocolate Avocado Mousse

Servings: 2 | Prep Time: 10 mins | Cooking Time: 25 mins

Ingredients:

- 2 ripe avocados
- 1/4 cup cocoa powder
- 1/4 cup honey or maple syrup
- 1 teaspoon vanilla extract
- Fresh berries for garnish (strawberries, raspberries)

Instructions:

- ✓ In a food processor, put together the avocados, cocoa powder, honey or maple syrup, and vanilla extract.
- ✓ Blend until everything is smooth.
- ✓ Chill in the refrigerator for thirty minutes.
- ✓ Serve topped with fresh berries.

Peanut Butter and Banana Smoothie

Servings: 2 | Prep Time: 5 mins | Cooking Time: 0 mins

Ingredients:

- 2 ripe bananas
- 2 tablespoons peanut butter

- 1 cup almond milk
- 1 tablespoon honey or maple syrup
- 1/2 teaspoon cinnamon

Instructions:

- ✓ In a blender, put together the bananas, peanut butter, almond milk, honey or maple syrup, and cinnamon.
- ✓ Blend until everything is smooth.
- ✓ Serve immediately.

Berry and Chia Seed Parfait

Servings: 2 | Prep Time: 10 mins | Freezing Time:120 mins

Ingredients:

- 1 cup mixed berries
- 1/4 cup Greek yogurt
- 2 tablespoons chia seeds
- 1 tablespoon honey or maple syrup

Instructions:

- ✓ In a jar or glass, layer mixed berries, Greek yogurt, chia seeds, and honey or maple syrup.
- ✓ Repeat the layers.
- ✓ Put in a refrigerator for at least two hours or overnight.

Baked Apples with Cinnamon and Walnuts

Servings: 2 | Prep Time: 10 mins | Cooking Time: 25 mins

Ingredients:

- 4 apples, cored and halved
- 1/4 cup chopped walnuts
- 1 tablespoon honey or maple syrup
- 1/2 teaspoon cinnamon
- Greek yogurt for topping (optional)

Instructions:

- ✓ Set the temperature of the oven to 375 degrees Fahrenheit (190 degrees Celsius).
- ✓ In a bowl, put together chopped walnuts, honey or maple syrup, and cinnamon.
- ✓ Fill each apple half with the mixture.
- ✓ Bake for twenty to twenty-five minutes.
- ✓ Serve with a dollop of Greek yogurt if desired.

Raspberry and Almond Oat Bars

Servings: 8 | Prep Time: 10 mins | Cooking Time: 25 mins

Ingredients:

- 1 cup rolled oats
- 1/2 cup almond butter
- 1/4 cup honey or maple syrup
- 1/4 cup dried raspberries
- 1/4 cup sliced almonds

Instructions:

- ✓ Set the temperature of the oven to 375 degrees Fahrenheit (190 degrees Celsius).
- ✓ In a bowl, put together the rolled oats, almond butter, honey or maple syrup, dried raspberries, and sliced almonds.
- ✓ Press the mixture into a lined baking pan.
- ✓ Bake for twenty to twenty-five minutes.
- ✓ Allow to cool before cutting into bars.

Grilled Pineapple with Coconut Yogurt

Servings: 4 | Prep Time: 10 mins | Cooking Time: 6 mins

Ingredients:

- 1 pineapple, peeled and sliced into rings
- 1 cup coconut yogurt
- 2 tablespoons honey or maple syrup
- Shredded coconut for garnish

Instructions:

- ✓ Set the temperature of the grill to moderate to high heat.
- ✓ Grill pineapple rings for two to three minutes per side until caramelized.
- ✓ In a bowl, put together the coconut yogurt and honey or maple syrup.
- ✓ Serve grilled pineapple with a dollop of coconut yogurt.
- ✓ Garnish with shredded coconut.

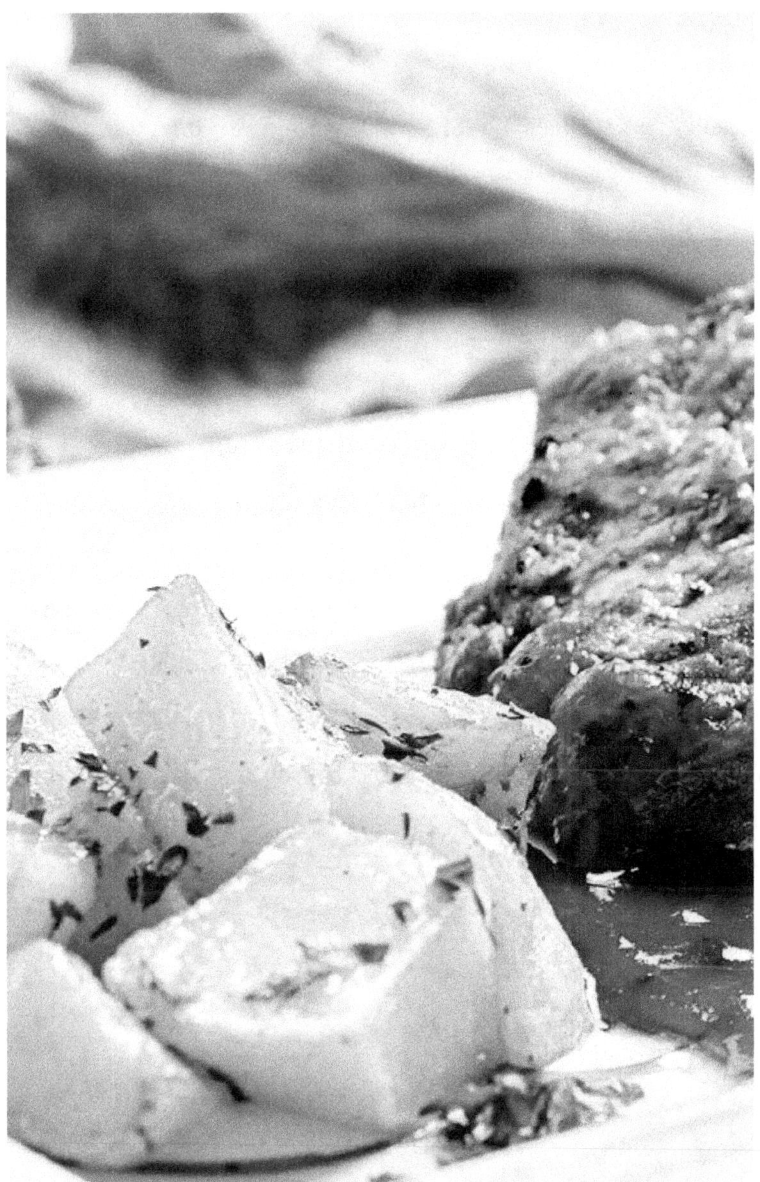

FRUITS AND DESSERTS

Berry Blast Smoothie Bowl

Servings: 1 | Prep Time: 5 mins | Cooking Time: 0 mins

Ingredients:

- 1 cup mixed berries
- 1 ripe banana
- 1/2 cup Greek yogurt
- 2 tablespoons honey or maple syrup
- Granola and sliced almonds for topping

Instructions:

- ✓ In a blender, put together the mixed berries, banana, Greek yogurt, and honey or maple syrup.
- ✓ Blend until everything is smooth.
- ✓ Transfer into a bowl and top with granola and sliced almonds.

Chocolate-Dipped Strawberries

Servings: 4 | Prep Time: 10 mins | Cooling Time:10 mins

Ingredients:

- 12 strawberries
- 4 oz dark chocolate, melted

Chopped nuts or shredded coconut for topping (optional)

Instructions:

- ✓ Line a baking sheet with parchment paper.
- ✓ Dip each strawberry into the melted dark chocolate.
- ✓ Place on the prepared sheet and sprinkle with chopped nuts or shredded coconut if desired.
- ✓ Allow to cool and harden.

Mango and Coconut Popsicles

Servings: 4 | Prep Time: 10 mins | Freezing Time: 240 mins

Ingredients:

- 2 ripe mangoes, peeled and diced
- 1 cup coconut milk
- 2 tablespoons honey or maple syrup

Instructions:

- ✓ In a blender, put together the diced mangoes, coconut milk, and honey or maple syrup.
- ✓ Blend until everything is smooth.
- ✓ Transfer into popsicle molds and freeze for at least four (4) hours.

Peanut Butter Banana Ice Cream

Servings: 2 | Prep Time: 10 mins | Cooking Time: 0 mins

Ingredients:

- 4 ripe bananas, sliced and frozen
- 2 tablespoons peanut butter
- 1/4 cup almond milk
- Dark chocolate chips for topping (optional)

Instructions:

- ✓ In a food processor, put together the frozen banana slices, peanut butter, and almond milk.
- ✓ Blend until everything is smooth.
- ✓ Serve immediately, topped with dark chocolate chips if desired.

Blueberry and Almond Chia Pudding

Servings: 2 | Prep Time: 5 mins | Freezing Time: 120 mins

Ingredients:

- 1/4 cup chia seeds

- 1 cup almond milk
- 1/2 cup fresh blueberries
- 2 tablespoons honey or maple syrup
- Sliced almonds for topping

Instructions:

- ✓ In a jar or bowl, put together the chia seeds, almond milk, blueberries, and honey or maple syrup.
- ✓ Stir very well.
- ✓ Refrigerate for at least two (2) hours or overnight.
- ✓ Top with sliced almonds before serving.

Pineapple and Coconut Sorbet

Servings: 4 | Prep Time: 5 mins | Freezing Time: 120 mins

Ingredients:

- 2 cups pineapple chunks
- 1/2 cup coconut milk
- 2 tablespoons honey or maple syrup

Instructions:

- ✓ In a blender, put together the pineapple chunks, coconut milk, and honey or maple syrup.
- ✓ Blend until everything is smooth.
- ✓ Transfer to a container and freeze for at least two (2) hours.

✓ Scoop and serve.

Apple and Cinnamon Oatmeal Cookies

Servings: 12 | Prep Time: 10 mins | Cooking Time: 20 mins

Ingredients:

- 2 cups rolled oats
- 2 ripe bananas, mashed
- 1 apple, grated
- 1/2 teaspoon cinnamon
- 1/4 cup honey or maple syrup
- 1/4 cup raisins or dried cranberries

Instructions:

✓ Set the temperature of the oven to 375 degrees Fahrenheit (190 degrees Celsius).

✓ In a bowl, put together the rolled oats, mashed bananas, grated apple, cinnamon, honey or maple syrup, and raisins or dried cranberries.

✓ Drop heaping spoonful of the mixture onto a baking sheet lined with parchment paper.

✓ Bake for fifteen to twenty minutes.

Mango and Pineapple Salsa

Servings: 4 | Prep Time: 10 mins | Cooking Time: 0 mins

Ingredients:

- 1 mango, peeled and diced
- 1 cup diced pineapple
- 1/4 cup red onion, finely chopped
- 1/4 cup fresh cilantro, chopped
- Juice of 1 lime
- Salt and pepper to taste

Instructions:

- ✓ In a bowl, put together the diced mango, diced pineapple, red onion, and cilantro.
- ✓ Squeeze lime juice over the top.
- ✓ Adjust with a little salt and pepper to your preferred taste.
- ✓ Serve as a salsa with tortilla chips or as a topping for grilled chicken or fish.

Strawberry and Almond Bites

Servings: 4 | Prep Time: 5 mins | Cooking Time: 0 mins

Ingredients:

- 1 cup strawberries, halved
- 1/4 cup almond butter
- 1/4 cup sliced almonds

Instructions:

- ✓ Spread almond butter onto each strawberry half.
- ✓ Sprinkle with sliced almonds.
- ✓ Serve as a snack or dessert.

Kiwi and Blueberry Parfait

Servings: 2 | Prep Time: 10 mins | Cooking Time: 0 mins

Ingredients:

- 2 kiwis, peeled and sliced
- 1 cup blueberries
- 1/4 cup Greek yogurt
- 2 tablespoons honey or maple syrup

Instructions:

✓ In a jar or glass, layer kiwi slices, blueberries, Greek yogurt, and honey or maple syrup.

✓ Repeat the layers.

✓ Serve immediately.

Chocolate Raspberry Chia Pudding

Servings: 2 | Prep Time: 5 mins | Freezing Time: 120 mins

Ingredients:

- 1/4 cup chia seeds
- 1 cup almond milk
- 1/4 cup cocoa powder
- 2 tablespoons honey or maple syrup
- 1/2 cup fresh raspberries

Instructions:

✓ In a jar or bowl, put together the chia seeds, almond milk, cocoa powder, and honey or maple syrup.

✓ Stir very well.

✓ Refrigerate for at least two (2) hours or overnight.

✓ Top with fresh raspberries before serving.

Watermelon and Mint Salad

Servings: 4 | Prep Time: 10 mins | Cooking Time: 0 mins

Ingredients:

- 4 cups cubed watermelon
- 1/4 cup fresh mint leaves, chopped
- Juice of 1 lime
- 1 tablespoon honey or maple syrup
- Feta cheese for topping (optional)

Instructions:

- ✓ In a bowl, put together the cubed watermelon and chopped fresh mint leaves.
- ✓ Squeeze lime juice over the top and drizzle with honey or maple syrup.
- ✓ Toss carefully and gently.
- ✓ Sprinkle with feta cheese if desired.

Grilled Peaches with Honey and Yogurt

Servings: 4 | Prep Time: 10 mins | Cooking Time: 6 mins

Ingredients:

- 4 ripe peaches, halved and pitted
- 1/4 cup honey
- Greek yogurt for topping
- Chopped pistachios for garnish

Instructions:

- ✓ Set the temperature of the grill to moderate to high heat.
- ✓ Grill peach halves for two to three minutes per side until caramelized.
- ✓ Drizzle with honey.
- ✓ Serve with a dollop of Greek yogurt and garnish with chopped pistachios.

30-DAY

MEAL

PLAN

<u>KEY</u>

A- BREAKFAST

B- LUNCH

C- DINNER

DAY	A	B	C
1	Oatmeal with sliced strawberries and almonds	Grilled chicken salad with spinach, avocado, and quinoa	Baked salmon with steamed broccoli and brown rice
2	Spinach and tomato omelet with whole-grain toast	Tuna salad sandwich on whole-grain bread with a side of carrot sticks	Turkey chili with mixed beans and a side salad
3	Berry and banana smoothie with Greek yogurt and chia seeds	Lentil soup with a whole-grain roll	Grilled shrimp skewers with quinoa and roasted vegetables
4	Oatmeal with walnuts, honey, and sliced strawberries	Whole-grain pasta with grilled vegetables and marinara sauce	Baked chicken breast, sweet potato, and green beans
5	Whole-grain pancakes with mixed berries and a side of Greek yogurt	Black bean and vegetable burrito bowl with brown rice	Stir-fried tofu with broccoli, bell peppers, and quinoa

DAY	A	B	C
6	Avocado toast with poached eggs and a side of mixed fruit	Turkey and avocado wrap with a side of raw veggies	Grilled cod with couscous and roasted Brussels sprouts
7	Chia seed pudding with almond milk and sliced peaches	Quinoa salad with mixed greens, cucumber, and grilled chicken	Baked turkey meatballs with whole-grain spaghetti and marinara sauce
8	Greek yogurt with honey, nuts, and mixed berries	Spinach and feta stuffed bell peppers with a side salad	Baked salmon with quinoa and steamed broccoli
9	Veggie scramble with mushrooms, onions, and bell peppers	Lentil and vegetable stew with a side of whole-grain bread	Grilled chicken stir-fry with brown rice and mixed vegetables
10	Whole-grain waffles with sliced bananas and Greek yogurt	Chickpea and vegetable curry with brown rice	Baked tilapia with quinoa salad and roasted Brussels sprouts

DAY	A	B	C
11	Berry smoothie bowl with granola and sliced almonds	Turkey and avocado sandwich on whole-grain bread with a side of carrot sticks	Beef and vegetable kebabs with brown rice
12	Whole-grain toast with avocado and scrambled eggs	Lentil and vegetable soup with a whole-grain roll	Baked chicken thighs with sweet potato and steamed asparagus
13	Greek yogurt parfait with mixed berries and nuts	Grilled vegetable and quinoa salad	Baked cod with couscous & roasted Brussels sprouts
14	Oatmeal with sliced strawberries and almonds	Black bean and vegetable burritos with a side of brown rice	Stir-fried tofu with broccoli and quinoa
15	Whole-grain pancakes with mixed berries and a side of Greek yogurt	Quinoa salad with mixed greens, cucumber, and grilled chicken	Baked turkey meatballs with whole-grain spaghetti and marinara sauce

DAY	A	B	C
16	Greek yogurt with honey, nuts, and mixed berries	Spinach and feta stuffed bell peppers with a side salad	Baked salmon with quinoa and steamed broccoli
17	Veggie scramble with mushrooms, onions, and bell peppers	Lentil and vegetable stew with a side of whole-grain bread	Grilled chicken stir-fry with brown rice and mixed vegetables
18	Whole-grain waffles with sliced bananas and Greek yogurt	Chickpea and vegetable curry with brown rice	Baked tilapia with quinoa salad and roasted Brussels sprouts
19	Berry smoothie bowl with granola and sliced almonds	Turkey and avocado sandwich on whole-grain bread with a side of carrot sticks	Beef and vegetable kebabs with brown rice
20	Whole-grain toast with avocado and scrambled eggs	Lentil and vegetable soup with a whole-grain roll	Baked chicken thighs with sweet potato and steamed asparagus

DAY	A	B	C
21	Greek yogurt parfait with mixed berries and nuts	Grilled vegetable and quinoa salad	Baked cod with couscous and roasted Brussels sprouts
22	Oatmeal with sliced strawberries and almonds	Black bean and vegetable burritos with a side of brown rice	Stir-fried tofu with broccoli and quinoa
23	Whole-grain pancakes with mixed berries and a side of Greek yogurt	Quinoa salad with mixed greens, cucumber, and grilled chicken	Baked turkey meatballs with whole-grain spaghetti and marinara sauce
24	Greek yogurt with honey, nuts, and mixed berries	Spinach and feta stuffed bell peppers with a side salad	Baked salmon with quinoa and steamed broccoli
25	Veggie scramble with mushrooms, onions, and bell peppers	Lentil and vegetable stew with a side of whole-grain bread	Grilled chicken stir-fry with brown rice and mixed vegetables

DAY	A	B	C
26	Whole-grain waffles with sliced bananas and Greek yogurt	Chickpea and vegetable curry with brown rice	Baked tilapia with quinoa salad and roasted Brussels sprouts
27	Berry smoothie bowl with granola and sliced almonds	Turkey and avocado sandwich on whole-grain bread with a side of carrot sticks	Beef and vegetable kebabs with brown rice
28	Whole-grain toast with avocado and scrambled eggs	Lentil and vegetable soup with a whole-grain roll	Baked chicken thighs with sweet potato and steamed asparagus
29	Greek yogurt parfait with mixed berries and nuts	Grilled vegetable and quinoa salad	Baked cod with couscous and roasted Brussels sprouts
30	Oatmeal with sliced strawberries and almonds	Black bean and vegetable burritos with a side of brown rice	Stir-fried tofu with broccoli and quinoa

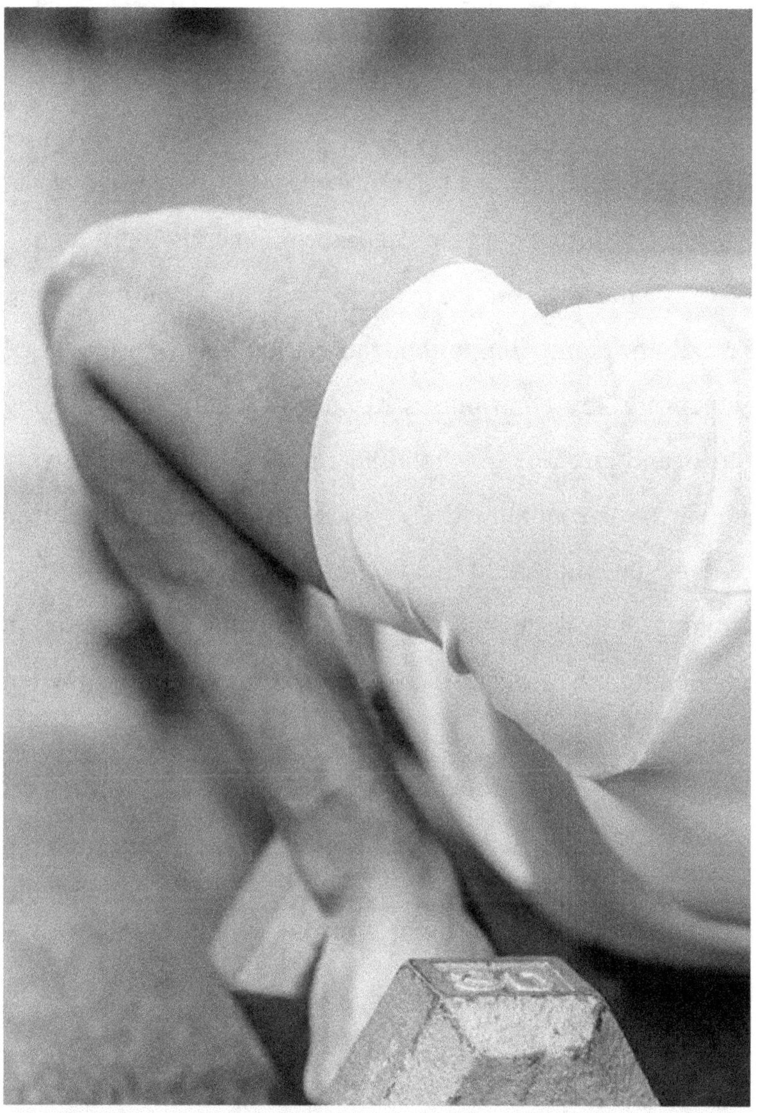

Simple Exercises to Boost Male Fertility & Improve Sexual Life

The Role of Exercise in Improving Male Fertility and Sperm Count

Regular physical activity plays an essential role in improving sperm count and overall reproductive health. Exercise helps to maintain a healthy weight, reduce inflammation, and enhance blood circulation, all of which are key contributors to better fertility. By reducing stress and improving general health, exercise can positively impact sperm count, which is essential for fertility. Scientific studies have indicated that activities such as weight-lifting, running, and jogging can potentially lead to higher sperm concentrations compared to other forms of exercise. When combined with a well-balanced and nutritious diet, regular exercise can naturally boost fertility levels. Therefore, embracing physical activities like hitting the gym, running, or any form of exercise that elevates your heart rate is highly beneficial.

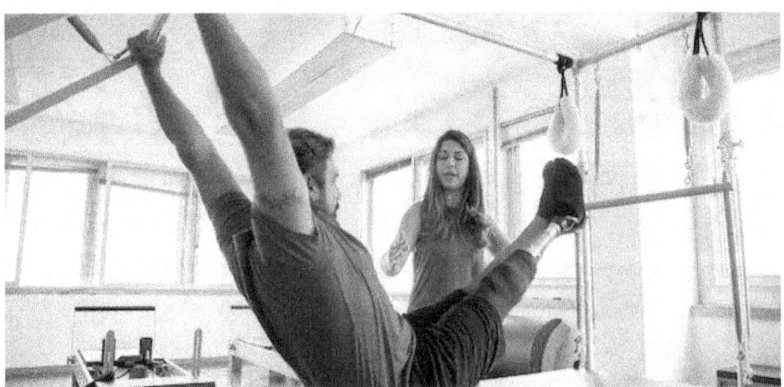

What Are the Top Exercises for Increasing Sperm Count and Boosting Male Fertility?

Cardiovascular Workouts

Engaging in cardiovascular exercises such as jogging, cycling, and swimming can greatly contribute to improved sperm quality and count. These activities effectively increase blood circulation throughout the body, including the reproductive organs, consequently enhancing the health of the testicles and promoting the production of healthier and more abundant sperm.

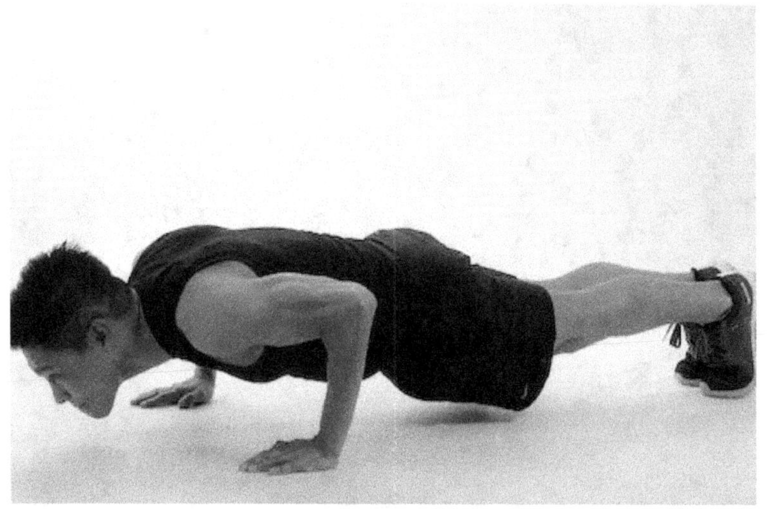

Resistance Training

Participating in resistance training, such as weight lifting and bodyweight workouts, can lead to increased testosterone levels in men. Testosterone is a fundamental hormone that plays a crucial role in sperm production. Elevated levels of testosterone can result in a higher sperm count. Incorporating compound exercises like squats and deadlifts into your workout routine can yield the best results.

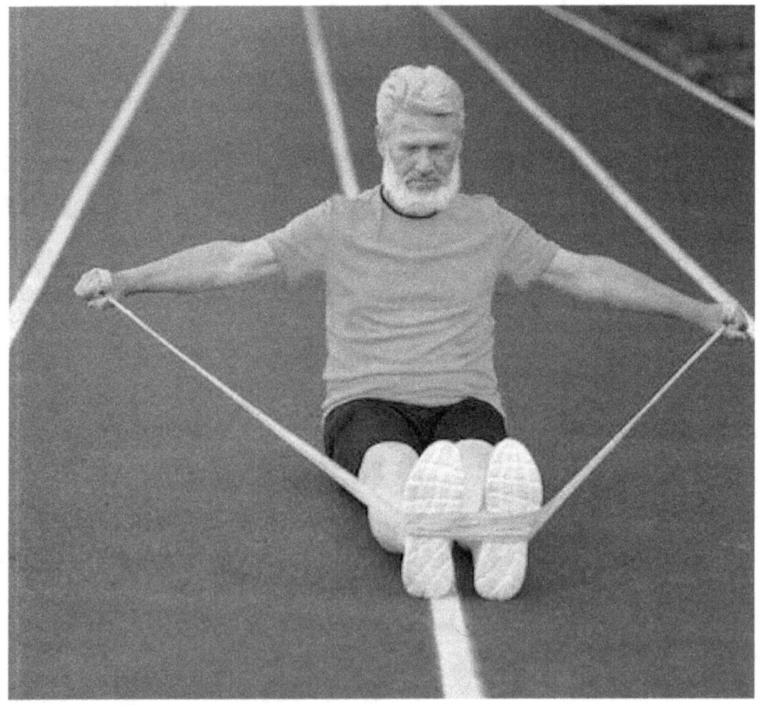

Yoga and Stress Reduction

High-stress levels can negatively affect fertility due to hormonal imbalances. Engaging in stress-reducing activities such as yoga, meditation, and relaxation techniques can help alleviate stress and anxiety, creating a healthier environment for sperm production.

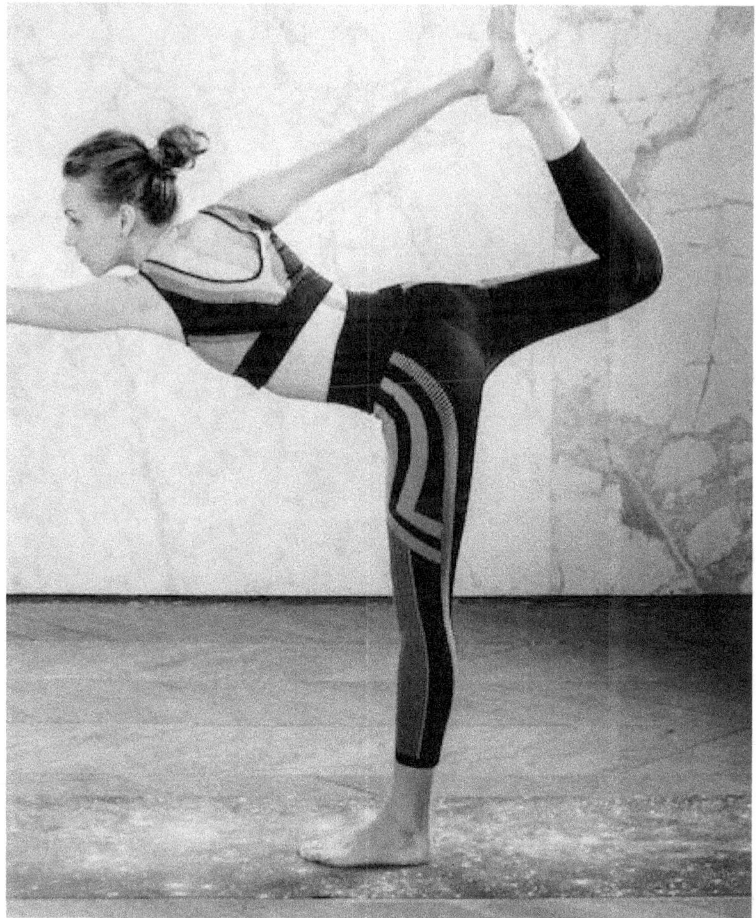

Kegel Exercises

Kegel exercises, beneficial for both men and women, focus on strengthening the pelvic floor muscles, which are essential for better sexual health. By improving ejaculation control and the strength of erections, Kegel exercises ultimately contribute to higher fertility levels.

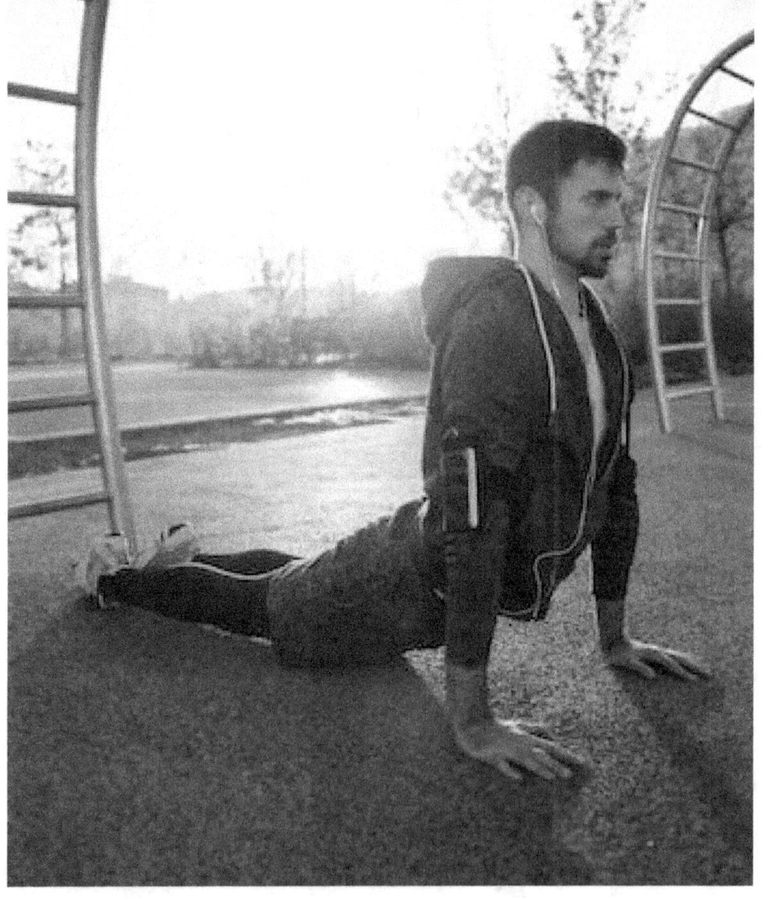

High Intensity Interval Training (HIIT)

High-intensity interval training (HIIT) has been shown to be an effective way to improve sperm count and fertility. HIIT workouts, involving short bursts of intense activity followed by brief rest periods, stimulate the production of testosterone, which is crucial for sperm production.

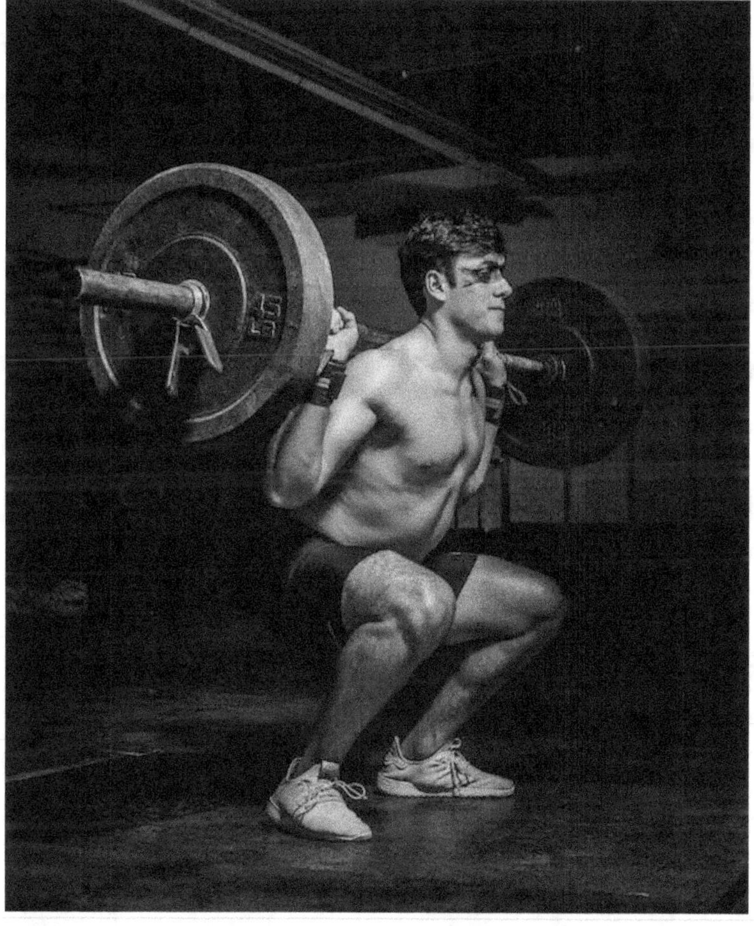

Aerobic Exercises

Participating in aerobic exercises such as aerobics classes or dancing is a fun way to boost sperm count and enhance cardiovascular health. These activities not only increase stamina and energy levels but also contribute to a healthy sex life and fertility.

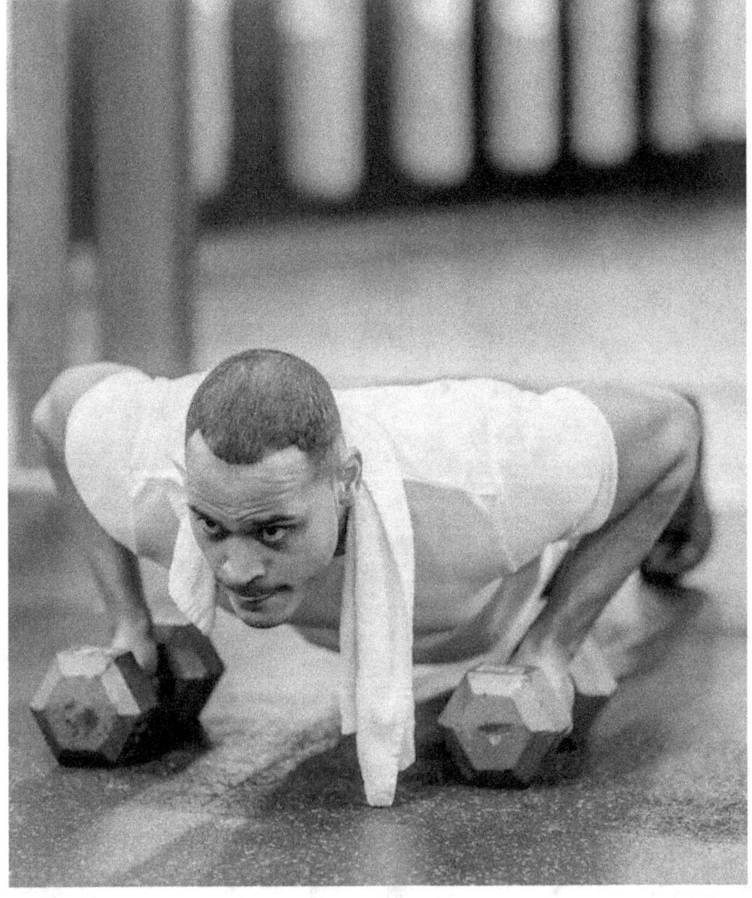

Swimming

Swimming is an exceptional full-body workout that can promote male fertility. Being a low-impact exercise, it does not place stress on the joints. Swimming on a regular basis can improve overall fitness and boost sperm count as time goes by.

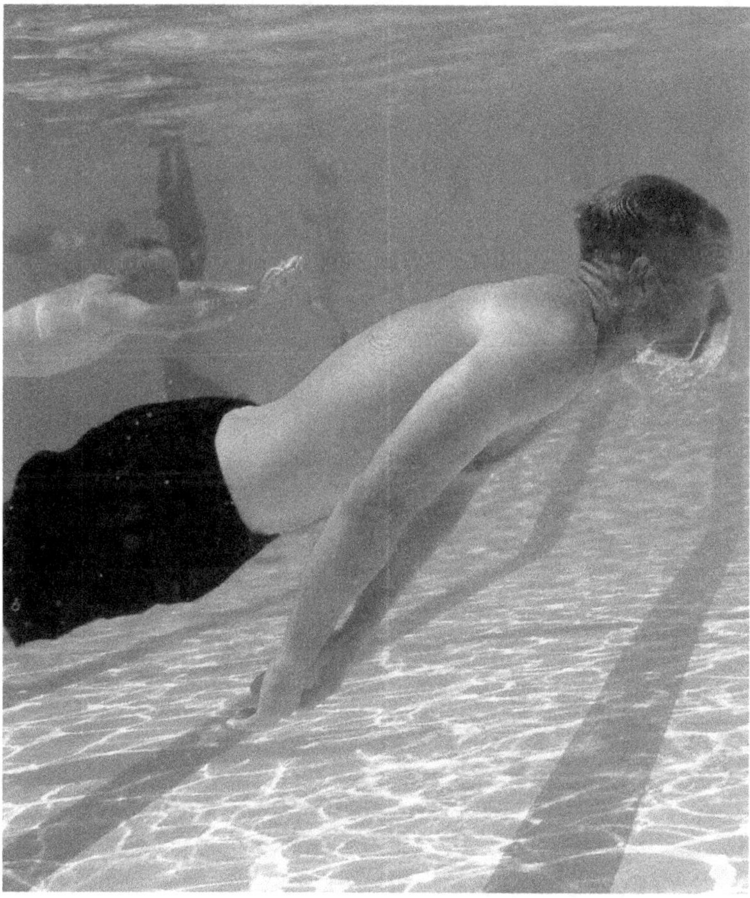

Pilates

Pilates, focusing on core strength and flexibility, plays an important role in sexual health. By improving core muscles and flexibility, Pilates can enhance sexual performance and potentially boost fertility.

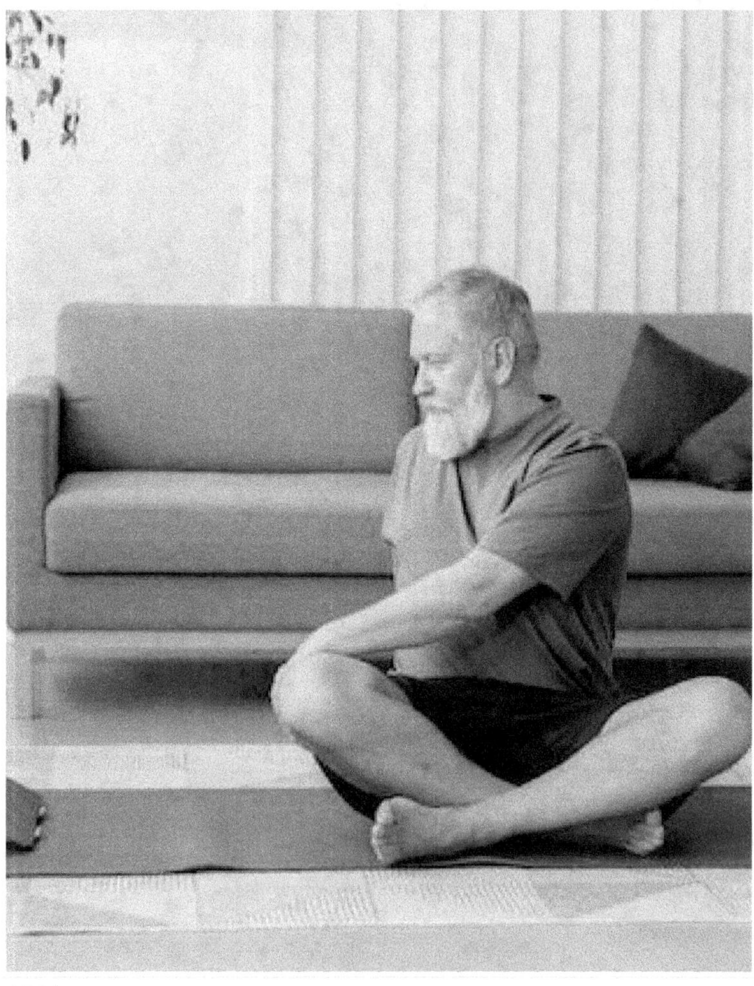

Cycling

While excessive cycling may have a negative impact on sperm count due to pressure on the perineum, moderate cycling can be beneficial. It is important to invest in a comfortable, well-fitted saddle to reduce pressure on the reproductive organs.

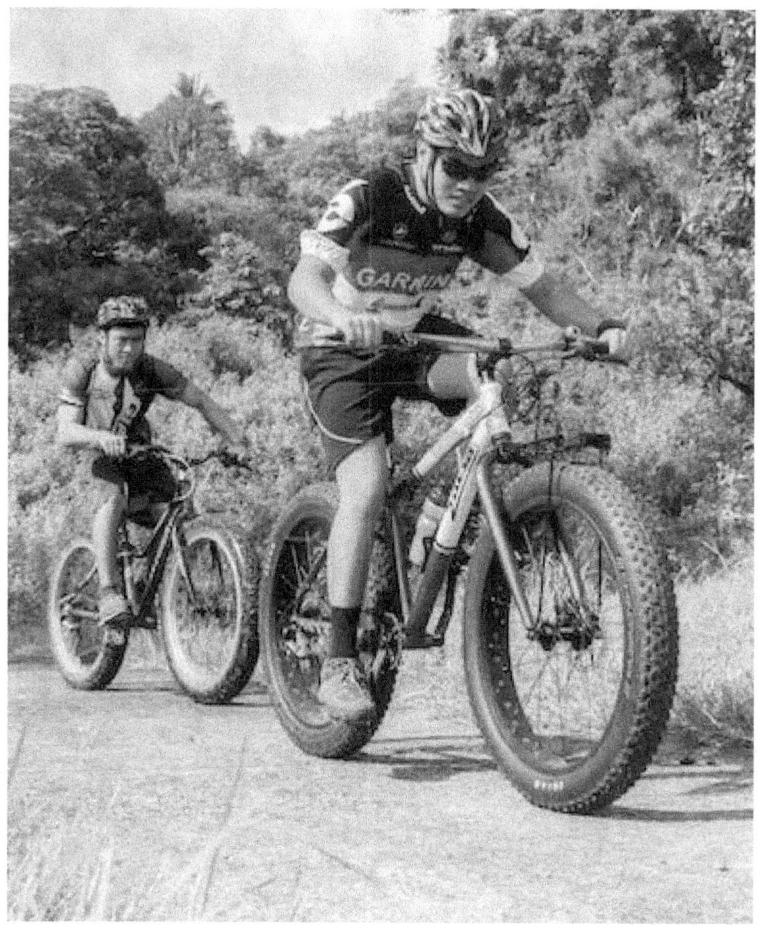

Tai Chi

Tai Chi, as a low-impact martial art that combines deep breathing and gentle movements, can help reduce stress levels and promote relaxation, creating a more favorable environment for sperm production.

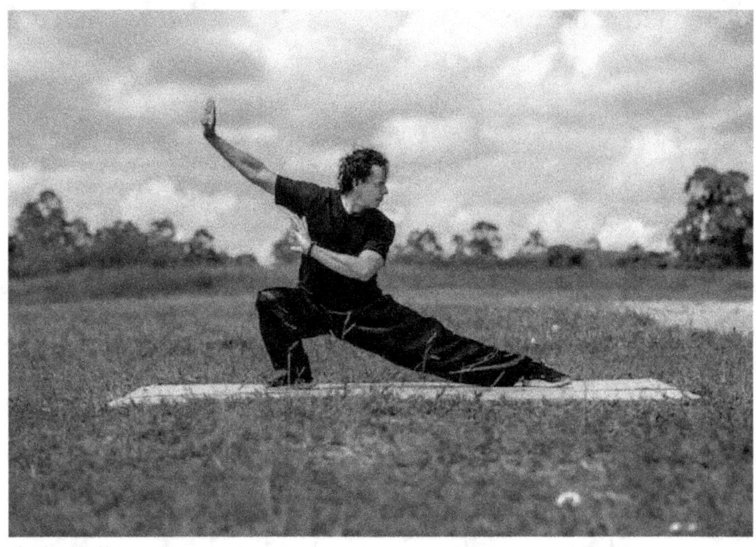

Adding a variety of exercises into your routine can significantly improve general health, reduce stress, and promote better reproductive health, ultimately leading to higher sperm count and improved fertility. Embracing physical activities that you enjoy and that elevate your heart rate can play a vital role in achieving better reproductive health.

Weekly Meal Planner

WEEKS	BREAKFAST	LUNCH	DINNER
MON			
TUE			
WED			
THU			
FRI			
SAT			
SUN			

Weekly Meal Planner

WEEKS	BREAKFAST	LUNCH	DINNER
MON			
TUE			
WED			
THU			
FRI			
SAT			
SUN			

Weekly Meal Planner

WEEKS	BREAKFAST	LUNCH	DINNER
MON			
TUE			
WED			
THU			
FRI			
SAT			
SUN			

Weekly Meal Planner

WEEKS	BREAKFAST	LUNCH	DINNER
MON			
TUE			
WED			
THU			
FRI			
SAT			
SUN			

Weekly Meal Planner

WEEKS	BREAKFAST	LUNCH	DINNER
MON			
TUE			
WED			
THU			
FRI			
SAT			
SUN			

Weekly Meal Planner

WEEKS	BREAKFAST	LUNCH	DINNER
MON			
TUE			
WED			
THU			
FRI			
SAT			
SUN			

Weekly Meal Planner

WEEKS	BREAKFAST	LUNCH	DINNER
MON			
TUE			
WED			
THU			
FRI			
SAT			
SUN			

Weekly Meal Planner

WEEKS	BREAKFAST	LUNCH	DINNER
MON			
TUE			
WED			
THU			
FRI			
SAT			
SUN			

NOTES

NOTES

NOTES

NOTES

NOTES

NOTES

NOTES

NOTES

NOTES

NOTES

www.ingramcontent.com/pod-product-compliance
Lightning Source LLC
Chambersburg PA
CBHW070941260726
48661CB00003B/1071